General Preface to the Series

It is no longer possible for one textbook to cover the whole field of Biology and to remain sufficiently up-to-date. At the same time teachers and students at school, college or university need to keep abreast of recent trends and know where the most significant developments are taking place.

To meet the need for this progressive approach the Institute of Biology has for some years sponsored this series of booklets dealing with subjects specially selected by a panel of editors. The enthusiastic acceptance of the series by teachers and students at school, college and university shows the usefulness of the books in providing a clear and up-to-date coverage of topics, particularly in areas of research and changing views.

Among features of the series are the attention given to methods, the inclusion of a selected list of books for further reading and, wherever possible, suggestions for practical work.

Readers' comments will be welcomed by the author or the Education Officer of the Institute.

1978   The Institute of Biology,
                                              41 Queens Gate,
                                              London, SW7 5HU

Preface

For many years the rat has served as a model animal for students of biology. Because it is a fairly characteristic animal, studies of its anatomy, physiology and behaviour provide reasonable insight into the general biology of mammals. What the rat has been to the zoologist, the haemoglobin molecule has become for students of molecular biology and biochemistry. It is a model molecule, and the student who understands the details of haemoglobin structure and function will not easily lose his way in the complex labyrinth of modern biochemistry.

Actually, haemoglobin is more than a good model. It has also served the pioneer researcher as a most valuable tool in many novel and illuminating experiments. In this small book I have therefore tried to use a discussion of haemoglobin to reveal both the elements of the molecular biology of proteins and some of the excitement of modern biological research.

I am most grateful to both my friend John Macfadyen for reading the text as a layman and to Professor D. J. Weatherall for reading it as an expert. Both have initiated several corrections and improvements.

1978   N. M.

Contents

The Institute of Biology's
Studies in Biology no. 93

Haemoglobin

Norman Maclean

Reader, department of biology,
University of Southampton

© Norman Maclean 1978

First published 1978
by Edward Arnold (Publishers) Limited
25 Hill Street, London W1X 8LL

Board edition ISBN: 0 7131 2697 3
Paper edition ISBN: 0 7131 2698 1

Printed in Great Britain by
The Camelot Press Ltd, Southampton

1 The Distribution and Physiology of Haemoglobin

1.1 **The distribution of haemoglobin and related molecules in living organisms**

Haemoglobin is widely known as the red pigment of vertebrate blood, but in fact its distribution is immensely wider than that statement suggests. Although not found in bacteria or any other prokaryotic cell, it occurs in such primitive nucleated cells as yeasts, some species of *Paramecium* and many invertebrate animals. Even plant cells are not left completely out of the picture since the root nodules of plants of the family Leguminosae contain a somewhat aberrant form of the molecule, termed leghaemoglobin. The uneven distribution of haemoglobin amongst invertebrates suggests that the molecule has evolved as an oxygen-carrying pigment more than once, prior to its final acceptance as the main oxygen carrier of vertebrate circulatory systems.

Let us, first of all, sketch its occurrence in the lower animals. It is commonly found in many Annelid worms, some nemerteans, many Crustacea (such as *Daphnia*, the water flea), a few insects and some Mollusca. In most of these organisms the pigment does not occur in blood cells but free in the haemolymph and is often of very high molecular weight. Its large size is accounted for simply by the aggregation of very many subunits to make one large polymeric molecule. Interestingly enough, haemoglobin is to be found within blood cells in a few invertebrates such as nemerteans and the mollusc *Arca*. Even the concentration of the pigment in specialized blood cells has therefore been anticipated early in evolution. But it must also be pointed out that in some of these lower organisms haemoglobin does not necessarily function as a respiratory pigment although it may always serve as an oxygen carrier. For example haemoglobin is found in the pharyngeal muscles of some snails and within the nerve cord of the sea mouse *Aphrodite* (an aberrant polychaete worm). In these sites the molecule no doubt serves the purpose of storing oxygen to prevent local anoxia, just as the related molecule myoglobin normally does in vertebrate muscle.

While we are discussing the distribution of haemoglobin in tissues and organisms, it is appropriate to briefly consider other molecules which living systems exploit as oxygen carriers (see Fig. 1–1). Haemoglobin is by no means the universal choice. Three other respiratory pigments occur sufficiently often in nature to deserve mention. The first is haemerythrin which is a form of haem, uncoupled with protein, operating as the sole respiratory pigment in a few marine worms. Chlorocruorin is a

Protein	Associated metal-prosthetic group	Distribution
(1) Myoglobin	Iron—haem	Muscle cells—widely distributed in animals from molluscs to man
(2) Haemoglobin	Iron—haem	Circulatory fluids—wide distribution in animals with exception of proto-chordates and most insects
(3) Haemocyanin	Copper—not linked to porphyrin	Circulatory fluids—molluscs and crustaceans
(4) Chlorocruorin	Iron—haem	Circulatory fluids—some annelid polychaete worms
(5) Haemerythrin	Iron—contains no porphyrins (nonhaem)	Circulatory fluids—some gephyrean annelids

Fig. 1–1 Examples of different types of respiratory proteins. (From Kagen, L. J. *Myoglobin*. Columbia Univ. Press, 1973.)

haem/protein complex closely similar to haemoglobin: the haem prosthetic group differs slightly. This molecule occurs as a respiratory pigment in many molluscs and worms, and some, such as the marine worm *Serpula*, possess both haemoglobin and chlorocruorin. Thirdly, many molluscs utilize an oxygen-carrying molecule based, not on iron, but on copper. Such molecules are termed haemocyanins.

We can therefore see that haemoglobin is a common but by no means the sole oxygen carrier in lower organisms. Even in the vertebrates it is not completely universal in its distribution. Two well-known examples of animals lacking haemoglobin are the young larvae of the common eel, and all stages of an antarctic fish known as the ice fish, illustrated in Fig. 1–2.

It is also important to remember that the distribution of haemoglobin has no direct relationship to the distribution of its prosthetic group, haem. The haem moiety contributes to the structure of cytochrome enzymes, catalases and peroxidases, as well as to myoglobin and haemoglobin. It follows that haem is to be found in the mitochondria of all animal and plant cells as well as in the cells of aerobic bacteria. The globin part of haemoglobin is normally assumed to be absent from organisms and tissues which lack haemoglobin, but we should admit that its presumed absence has rarely been checked.

By way of rounding off our discussion of respiratory pigments and

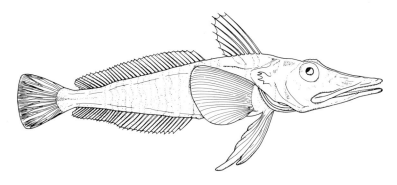

Fig. 1–2   The ice fish *Chaenocephalus aceratus*, an antarctic fish which entirely lacks haemoglobin. It attains a length of about 60 cm.

their distribution in nature, we should say a word about myoglobin. This molecule is found in vertebrate muscle, being particularly concentrated in red muscle to which the respiratory pigment provides its characteristic colour. Myoglobin is not so much an oxygen carrier as an oxygen storage molecule in muscle. It occurs as a single monomer combining a haem group with a globin protein. The globin, although distinct from those found in haemoglobin, is sufficiently similar to the globin chain of human haemoglobin to suggest that both proteins are the products of genes which may be derived from one ancestral globin gene.

1.1.1   Intracellular and extracellular haemoglobin

In many simple organisms no special respiratory circulation is required, since adequate oxygen is obtained by the cells by simple diffusion. Thus most insects, nematodes and jelly-fishes, to take a few obvious examples, rely on oxygen and carbon dioxide diffusion to accomplish gas exchange between their cells and the outer environment. The next stage in evolutionary sophistication comes with the increase in size and complexity of the organism, and here we first encounter a circulatory system and the need for an oxygen-carrying molecule. But at first the haemoglobin, or other oxygen-carrier, is simply in solution in the circulating fluid and indeed in some invertebrates there is circulation of dissolved oxygen without the help of a specific carrier molecule. Placement of the oxygen-carrying molecule within specialized blood cells occurs in a few invertebrates such as nemerteans, and some molluscs and echinoderms. In these animals the intracellular haemoglobin is of rather low molecular weight, which makes an interesting contrast to the enormous complexes of haemoglobin which circulate freely and extracellularly in more primitive invertebrates. Why, then, has the intracellular haemoglobin become the persistent theme of vertebrate circulation? The answer is chiefly one of efficient concentration and circulation. If haemoglobin was carried free in the circulating blood fluid, these large molecules would render the fluid highly viscous and difficult to circulate. By concentrating the molecules within cellular packages the overall viscosity is reduced. The blood corpuscles, nucleated in most vertebrates but non-nucleated in mammals, are sufficiently small to be squeezed through the fine capillaries which ramify through the tissues. It is always fascinating to study the blood circulation in the thin webbing of a living frog's foot by viewing, with transmitted light, through a low-power microscope. Each pumping stroke of the heart sends the oval flattened corpuscles further on their route, the cells forcing their way through blood vessels little wider (and sometimes narrower) than their own diameter.

It is also pertinent to consider here the respiratory problem which vertebrates would face if they lacked an oxygen-carrying molecule. If a man lacked haemoglobin and was forced to carry dissolved oxygen in simple aqueous solution, he would require a blood volume thirty times greater, or to circulate the same volume some thirty times faster. This then is some measure of our debt to the efficiency of the respiratory pigment, a thought which brings us naturally to the next consideration, the physiological characteristics of haemoglobin.

1.2 The association of haemoglobin with oxygen

Haemoglobin has several fascinating properties which relate to its ability to combine with oxygen. Basically the molecule functions by absorbing oxygen where the oxygen tension is high and releasing oxygen where the tension is low. By oxygen tension is meant the comparative pressure or concentration of oxygen prevailing in a solution. It is the ferrous iron atom in the haem nucleus to which the oxygen actually joins, but the globin part of the haemoglobin also plays a vital function in that oxygen does not combine reversibly with the haem group on its own, but only when it is complexed to globin. If, for the moment, we think of all haemoglobins as monomeric molecules consisting of one haem combined to one globin (as are, for example, the haemoglobins of lampreys and some hag fishes), we can more easily discuss the first aspect of oxygen association. When such a monomeric molecule is exposed to a high oxygen tension its haem group will absorb one atom of oxygen. This bound oxygen will remain attached to the haemoglobin monomer provided that the surrounding oxygen tension remains high. But if the haemoglobin is transported to a situation where oxygen tension is low, the bond becomes unstable and it will release the oxygen from the haem group. This, in simple terms, explains how oxygen is transported from the vertebrate lung, where tension is high, to the distant tissue cells, where it is much lower. The curve of this simple association between haemoglobin and oxygen would be hyperbolic, as shown in Fig. 1–3,

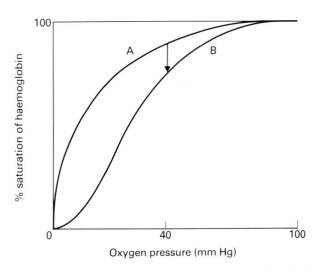

Fig. 1–3 Haemoglobin oxygen dissociation curves showing hyperbolic (A) and sigmoid (B) dissociation curves. When the pigment operates between an oxygen pressure of 100 and 40 mm Hg the length of the arrow represents the increased efficiency of a sigmoid curve. (From Lehmann, H. and Huntsman, R. G. *Man's Haemoglobins*. North Holland, 1974.)

implying that the oxygen would combine with all the haemoglobin molecules even at fairly low tensions but would also be discharged very readily at tensions only slightly lower. In other words the haemoglobin would easily become saturated but would readily give up its oxygen, often before it had reached situations of real oxygen demand.

The great breakthrough in improving the efficiency of haemoglobin as a carrier of oxygen comes with the properties of haemoglobin polymers. If dimers or tetramers of the simple haem and globin monomer are produced, it frequently follows that the oxygen uptake curve of one of the monomers is modified by the attachment of an oxygen atom to the other. (In this terminology a monomer is a single unit, a dimer two, tetramer four and polymer many.) When four monomers are grouped to form a tetramer, as they are in most vertebrate haemoglobins, then the oxygen tensions at which the molecular complex will accept or discharge oxygen come to be greatly stretched, yielding a sigmoid (S shaped) rather than a hyperbolic (shaped ⌡ or ⌐)) dissociation curve (see Fig. 1–3.) This sigmoid curve is of the utmost importance in vertebrate physiology, for it permits animals to bind and release oxygen over a wide range of oxygen concentrations. Moreover, different animals further exploit their haemoglobins by shifting the sigmoid curve up or down the gradient of oxygen concentration, depending on their way of life. Thus fish which live in stagnant waters have the curve moved to the left, so making oxygen capture from the water easier and oxygen release to the tissues occurring at lower tensions. On the other hand, fish living in regions rich in oxygen have their curves shifted to the right.

We have not as yet explained how a sigmoid dissociation curve is ever obtained; or, to put it in another way, how co-operation between haemoglobin monomers can actually modify their individual oxygen binding characteristics. The explanation lies in a phenomenon known as *allostery*, which is a change in shape and altered properties following from a molecule binding another at one of its active sites (see Fig. 1–4). When a single haem in a tetrameric haemoglobin molecule binds an oxygen atom, not only does the monomer with the bound oxygen change shape slightly, but this movement also alters the architecture of the whole complex. Further shifts occur when subunits two and three also bind oxygen, so that the last haem group has startlingly different oxygen

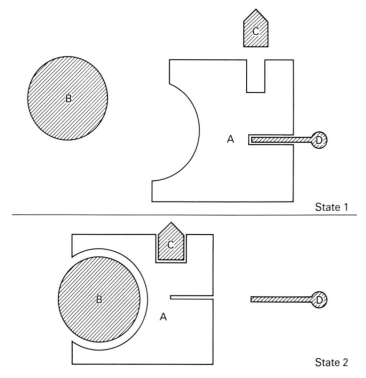

Fig. 1–4 Diagram to illustrate allostery. In State 1, the molecule A is not coupled with molecule B at the appropriate attachment site, thus permitting attachment of molecule D but excluding C. However, in State 2, on attachment of molecule B, the shape of A changes, thus excluding D but permitting attachment of C.

association characteristics from the first. The physical movement involved in haemoglobin allostery is relatively tiny, the subunits moving together by only a few Ångstrom units (an Ångstrom is 0.1 nanometres, i.e. there are 10 million Ångstroms in a millimetre) as each oxygen is bound. But this movement so alters the binding characteristics that the last haem group acquires an affinity for oxygen some hundreds of times greater than that of the first. The sigmoid curve also applies to oxygen release, so that the first oxygen atom is given up to the tissues very readily, but each succeeding oxygen atom with increasing difficulty and at greatly reduced oxygen tensions. The oxygenation of mammalian haemoglobin can therefore be represented as a four-step process:

$$Hb + O_2 \longrightarrow HbO_2$$
$$HbO_2 + O_2 \longrightarrow HbO_4$$
$$HbO_4 + O_2 \longrightarrow HbO_6$$
$$HbO_6 + O_2 \longrightarrow HbO_8$$

1.3   Factors affecting the oxygen uptake curve

The sigmoid curve representing association and dissociation of oxygen and haemoglobin is itself affected by a number of factors, some of which we will now discuss.

1.3.1   The nature of the globin polypeptide chain

We have already mentioned that the haem group itself is affected in its oxygen binding by the globin, and that indeed it will only effectively bind oxygen when conjugated to globin. Most vertebrate haemoglobins are tetramers with at least two different types of subunit, and this subunit complexity accounts for much of the allosteric association curves. Tetramers made artificially from one type of subunit only display a little allostery and have an essentially hyperbolic association curve. Moreover, as we will discuss at length in Chapter 2, many different globins may be synthesized in any one animal either at the same time or at different times. So most vertebrates possess different types of haemoglobin tetramers with different properties at different developmental stages. These may also coexist in the red cells in adult life. This endows the adult vertebrate with the potential of efficient respiration in a wide range of environmental conditions.

1.3.2   The Bohr effect

An important modulator of haemoglobin function is found in the hydrogen ion concentration of the cell. This is normally expressed as pH, and its effect on the oxygen/haemoglobin affinity is known as the Bohr effect, following its discovery by the Swedish physiologist of that name. For the majority of haemoglobins the relationship is direct, in that

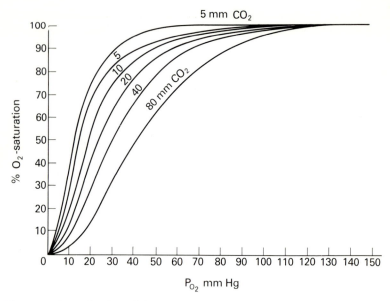

Fig. 1–5 Reproduction of the original graph by Bohr, Hasselbalch and Krogh (1904) demonstrating the effect of P_{CO_2} upon the O_2–affinity of human blood (the Bohr effect). Ordinate: percentage O_2-saturation; abscissa: P_{O_2}; temperature: 37°C. (From Steen, J. B. *Comparative Physiology of Respiratory Mechanisms*. Academic Press, 1971.)

reduction in pH leads to reduction in oxygen affinity (see Fig. 1–5). One of the important and fascinating results of the Bohr effect is that an increased CO_2 concentration in a vertebrate tissue leads to reduction in pH and consequent reduction in the affinity of the oxygen for the haemoglobin. In other words oxygen is released more readily by haemoglobin in tissues with an already high CO_2 content. A very useful device!

1.3.3 The Root effect

In 1931 the British biologist Root discovered that hydrogen ion concentration not only affected the *rate* of association with oxygen but also, in some cases, the *capacity* of the haemoglobin for oxygen-carrying. At high pH the oxygen capacity is increased and vice versa (see Fig. 1–6). The Bohr effect may occur in some species without any apparent Root effect, but a large Root effect always implies an accompanying high Bohr effect. The extent of both of these interesting phenomena varies with different animal species and different habitats.

1.3.4 Low molecular weight metabolites

The levels of some low molecular weight metabolites within the

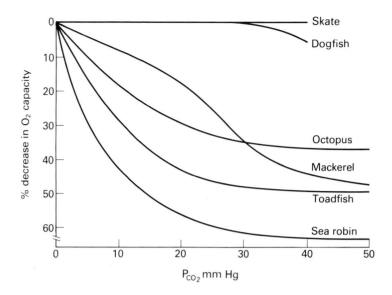

Fig. 1–6 The Root effect of blood from various fishes. (From Steen, J. B. *Comparative Physiology of Respiratory Mechanisms*. Academic Press, 1971.)

erythrocytes may also affect haemoglobin/oxygen affinity. One of the best known examples is that of 2,3-diphosphoglycerate (2,3-DPG) concentration and affinity in mammalian erythrocytes, oxygen affinity being reduced as concentrations of 2,3-DPG rise. It is now known that the exchange of oxygen between fetal and maternal blood cells across the human placental barrier at pregnancy is explained in this way. Although human adult and fetal haemoglobins differ, their uptake curves are similar, but the human fetal erythrocyte has a markedly lower 2,3-DPG affinity than its adult counterpart, thus permitting the oxygen transfer.

Human adaptation to high altitude also involves changes in the 2,3-DPG concentration within the erythrocyte. Of course, adaptation to altitude is a complex reaction in itself and some animal species, apparently excluding man, however, can compensate by synthesizing different haemoglobins with higher oxygen affinities. The commonest reaction of vertebrates to high altitude is simply an increase in the number of circulating erythrocytes, so stepping up the oxygen-carrying potential of the blood. But in addition it has been observed that during the first two days of exposure to altitudes in excess of 18 000 ft., an increase in the 2,3-DPG concentration occurs in the circulating erythrocytes. This interesting adaptation has the effect of easing the release of oxygen from the haemoglobin to the tissues.

1.3.5   The effect of temperature

Since haemoglobin can in many ways be regarded as an enzyme, some appreciation of enzyme kinetics and biochemistry will help us to understand the reactions of haemoglobin. But where most enzymic reactions are expressed in terms of the Michaelis Constant, K_M, it is useful to measure reactions involving haemoglobin in terms of the P_{50} value, which is the concentration of oxygen required to half saturate the Hb under given controlled conditions of pH, ionic strength and temperature. Now this leads us to the point that, as with other enzymes, the oxygen/Hb-reaction is greatly affected by temperature, but, interestingly enough, the direction of this temperature dependent effect is the opposite of what we might casually predict, or indeed what would be most obviously useful to the organism. In short, the P_{50} *increases* as temperature increases, implying that with increased temperature the Hb will find it harder to acquire the oxygen molecules. When we combine this knowledge with the appreciation that the amount of gas, e.g. oxygen, dissolved in water is inversely proportional to temperature, we can see that any animal trying to derive oxygen from warm water is in difficulties. Thus the immense fish populations in the cold polar seas and the not infrequent mass deaths of fresh water fish in inland waters during hot summers. What then can organisms do to counteract these dual difficulties? There seems little doubt that many species simply reduce their metabolism and become very sluggish, but species which are regularly exposed to rather rapid fluctuations in water temperature have often made a more strategic adaptation: they possess multiple haemoglobins with very differing oxygen affinities, and in very warm water the haemoglobin with the lowest P_{50} will be utilized chiefly. The possession of multiple types of haemoglobin, and their significance in development and evolution, will be discussed at greater length in the next chapter.

1.4   Carbon dioxide transport

Carbon dioxide is a much more soluble gas than oxygen and most of the carbon dioxide released by body cells during metabolism is transported to the lungs dissolved in the blood plasma. Some, however, is transported by haemoglobin due to the formation of carbaminohaemoglobin. So, although animals do not rely heavily on haemoglobin as a carrier of carbon dioxide, it does carry out this function to a small extent. And of course haemoglobin will also combine very readily with other gases: its preferential and highly stable association with carbon monoxide confers on this gas its highly lethal quality.

2   Haem and Globin—the Structure of Haemoglobin and its Variations

The haemoglobin molecule has a composite structure. Not only do the distinct haem and globin units combine to form the haemoglobin itself, but most, though not all, naturally occurring haemoglobins comprise aggregates of these single haemoglobin monomers. Most frequently four monomers are associated together to form the functional complex which we term haemoglobin, and commonly these monomers are of two distinct types so that the complete tetramer consists of two of one monomer type and two of another (see Fig. 2–1).

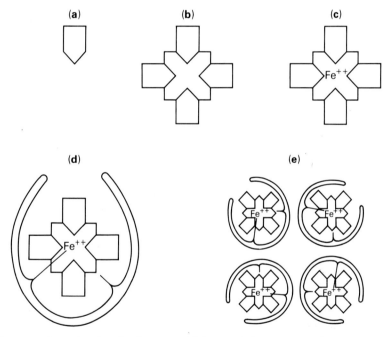

Fig. 2–1   Steps in the development of haemoglobin. a: pyrrole unit; b: porphyrin ring; c: haem; d: haem-globin complex (e.g. myoglobin); e: four haem-globin units forming one complex molecule (e.g. haemoglobin). (From Lehmann, H. and Huntsman, R. G. *Man's Haemoglobins*. North Holland, 1974.)

We can now discuss the actual structure of haemoglobin and its constituent parts, first by looking at the structure of haem and then of globin, then considering the monomer of one haem bonded to one globin, and finally the structure of the complete tetramer. The variations in the structures can be usefully remarked upon as we deal with each level of structure.

2.1   The structure of the haem group

Haem, alternatively spelled heme, constitutes the prosthetic group of the haemoglobin molecule. It is actually more correctly termed protohaem, and is a very stable coordination compound of iron and protoporphyrin IX. The structure of haem is illustrated in Fig. 2–2. There

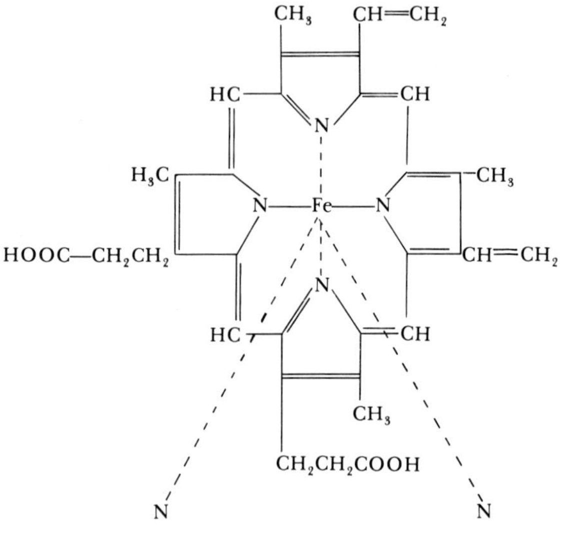

Fig. 2–2   The chemical structure of the haem group associated with each Hb polypeptide chain (subunit). The structure illustrates the state of the unit in deoxyhaemoglobin.

are fifteen possible isomeric forms of protoporphyrin, made possible by substitution of its propionic acid, vinyl and methyl residues, but only form IX is utilized in the formation of haem and is indeed the only isomer important in biology. Haems other than protohaem are found in some classes of cytochrome enzymes and are variously styled as haem A, a_2, and b. The iron atom in haem or protohaem is in the ferrous state (Fe^{2+}), but compounds also exist in which the iron is in the ferric state (Fe^{3+}). The molecule is then styled haematin, or hemin. As mentioned in Chapter 3, porphyrins may also be found in nature linked to metals other than iron. Thus the copper-containing haemocyanins, and the magnesium-based molecule chlorophyll.

Having sorted out this somewhat cumbersome terminology, let us return to our study of the structure of protohaem, which we will henceforward call, simply, haem. As we have stated, it is a ferrous iron atom combined to a porphyrin molecule. Reference to Fig. 2-2 will indicate at a glance that the iron atom is coupled to the porphyrin ring at four sites, each of these being a nitrogen atom. The iron also makes two other links, one being to the globin polypeptide chain (invariably to a histidine residue in the chain) and one to the oxygen atom being carried. If no oxygen is carried the sixth bonding position may be occupied by a water molecule. Of course physical chemistry now tells us that not only are atoms comprised of particles in a state of flux, with electrons orbiting about a central nucleus, but that electrons display a spinning motion which is related to the particular tracks which they follow round the atomic nucleus. The iron atom, whether in the ferric or ferrous state, can exist in different forms, these forms differing in the ways in which the electrons occupy the outer orbital shell. Of these, one is termed high spin and the other low spin, and the precise fit of the iron into the porphyrin ring affects the spin state. In the low spin state the iron atom fits snugly within the quadrangle of nitrogens, but in the high spin state the iron lies slightly outside the plane of the four nitrogen atoms. Oxygen serves as a ligand, or complexing agent, and its complex with the iron atom has two highly important characteristics. The first is that the ligand site only becomes operative when the iron of the haem is already complexed to the histidine residue of the globin chain, in other words that haem alone is not an effective oxygen carrier. The second is that when oxygen combines with haem as a ligand, it alters the spin state of the iron atom electrons: other molecules which may act as ligands, such as cyanide or carbon monoxide, also affect the spin state, but not always in the same way. What follows from the altered spin state of the iron atom accounts for the remarkable properties of the haemoglobin molecule. This is because the alteration in electron spin affects the fit of the iron in the porphyrin ring, which in turn affects the tertiary structure of the protein part of the haemoglobin monomer. As we shall see shortly, this accommodating change in shape on the part of the globin, following from the attachment of an oxygen atom, is used by the haemoglobin tetramer complex to accomplish its fascinating physiological properties.

The other special property of the haem group of respiratory protein is that, when oxygen is bound, the iron atom itself is not oxidized. Ferroprotoporphyrin itself will bind oxygen but the ferrous iron is rapidly oxidized to the ferric state and the molecule becomes functionally useless as an oxygen carrier. The critical property of retaining the iron atom in the ferrous state following association with oxygen also depends on the linkage between haem and globin. If the globin is denatured the property is lost.

2.2   The structure of globin

The globin portion of haemoglobin is a protein, and so we will now outline the general structure of these extremely important biological molecules. In general, proteins are constructed from linear, covalently bonded chains of small molecules termed amino acids. Since there are only about twenty different kinds of amino acids used in the structure of most proteins, we might imagine that the possible variety of proteins is small. But quite the opposite is the case. A protein consisting of a string of 100 amino acids (and many are much longer) can be assembled in 20^{100} different ways, each yielding a structurally unique molecule. So there are virtually no limits on the numbers of different kinds of proteins possible. The actual number is, no doubt, much smaller.

Since the bonds between amino acids are termed peptide linkages, the linear chain of amino acids is termed a polypeptide chain. It has become conventional to reserve the actual word protein for polypeptide chains of at least about 30 amino acids. So all proteins are polypeptide chains but not all polypeptide chains are properly styled proteins. We will begin our analysis of protein structure by thinking about the structure of the building blocks, the amino acids themselves.

2.2.1   Amino acid structure

In general amino acids are molecules with a molecular weight of about 100 to 200 and with the general formula NH_2—CHR—$COOH$, R being variable and often a side chain. The presence of the NH_2, known as the *amino* group, confers on proteins their important possession of nitrogen, and the $COOH$ configuration is known as the *carboxyl* group. As we shall see later, both groups are important in joining amino acids together to form proteins. Apart from the simplest of the amino acids, glycine, which has the formula H_2N—CH_2—$COOH$ (where R = H), all amino acids may exist in either D or L forms; that is, mirror images of the molecules can exist which will rotate polarized light in either the dextro (right) or laevo (left) direction. This is a consequence of the so-called α-carbon atom in the centre of the molecule being asymmetric and giving the molecule two alternative stable positional forms which are mirror images of each other. Although both D and L forms of most amino acids occur in cells, only the L forms are utilized in the structure of proteins. This astonishing observation has two significant aspects. One is that polypeptides of mixed D and L forms would be inherently unstable because of the inadequate positioning for peptide bond formation. The other is perhaps the more curious, namely that the L form has come to be the universal choice of living systems. One can perhaps spend a usefully cerebral weekend thinking of the possible biochemical and physiological consequences of having a totally D-form world, or, even more interesting, a world of organisms, some based on L amino acids and some based on D amino acids, both inherently incompatible! The selection of L-form amino acids must have been one of the first crucial choices in the evolutionary development of the first living cell.

2.2.2   The peptide linkage

When the elements of water are removed from the respective carboxyl and amino groups of two adjacent amino acids, we achieve a peptide linkage between them (see Fig. 2–3). Such a compound is a dipeptide. By continuing the process we produce polypeptides.

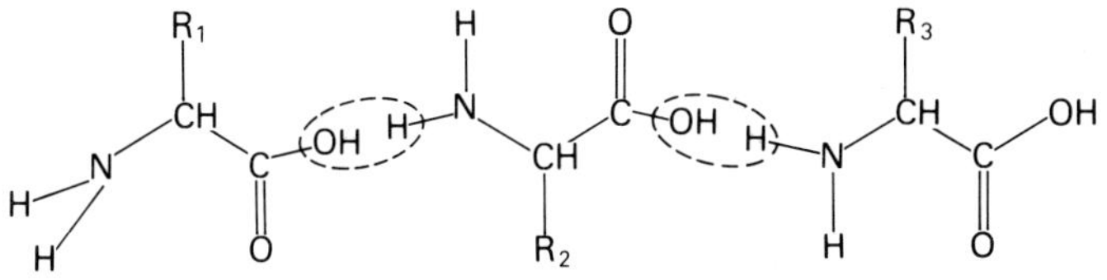

Three amino acids aligned to show the water molecule,
the elimination of which permits the peptide bond to form.

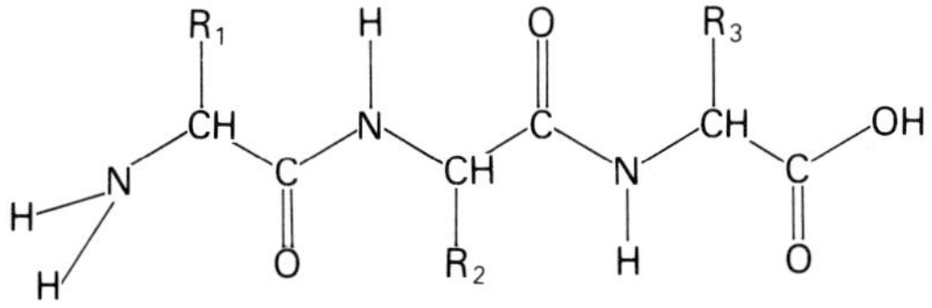

The same amino acids joined to form a tripeptide by
elimination of water

Fig. 2–3   The formation of peptide bonds by the elimination of water from two adjacent amino acids.

2.2.3   The structure of proteins

Although we have defined proteins as being simply polypeptide chains made up of strings of amino acids, they are, in fact, somewhat more complicated. They have indeed four different levels of structure which will be examined in turn.

Primary structure. This is simply the basic number and arrangement of amino acids in the polypeptide chain. For globins the number is around 150 amino acids in each monomer globin (see Fig. 2–4). The number itself varies with the different globins, being 141 for human α chain globin, and

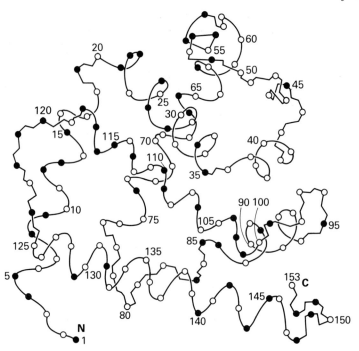

Fig. 2–4 Polypeptide structure of sperm whale myoglobin. Variant positions are shown by filled-in circles; positions constant among mammals studied thus far are indicated by open circles. (From Kagen, L. J. *Myoglobin*. Columbia Univ. Press, 1973.)

146 for human β chain globin and human γ chain globin. Myoglobin possesses 153 amino acid residues, while animal globins have numbers which are variable but roughly similar. We will discuss some of the significance of the similarities and differences in Chapter 4; it will suffice for us to comment at the moment that where groups of amino acids in the sequence remain unchanged in the course of evolution, we can predict that that part of the molecule has a particularly crucial function: that is, it is an active site. If we compare human α and β globins, 61 pairs of amino acids are identical (42% of the 146 residues), and some of these amino acids are unchanged even when very many different globin types are compared—for example the highly important histidine residue which is number 87 in the globin chain and which links to the iron atom of the haem group to form the haemoglobin monomer. (Polypeptide chains are, by convention, enumerated from a start at the free amino end of the molecule, termed the N-terminus: the other end is the C-terminus.)

Secondary structure. The next order of protein architecture is referred to as secondary structure, and this dimension refers to the basic configuration which the polypeptide chain adopts once the amino acids have been strung together. The structure is almost invariably a simple coil or helix and is referred to as the α helix. Each turn of the helix involves a length of about four amino acids. The α helix is normally stabilized by some bonding between amino acids lying above or below each other in adjacent turns. Not all parts of a polypeptide chain are in the form of a helix. As seen in Fig. 2–5, parts of the globin polypeptide chain in myoglobin are simply strung out and uncoiled.

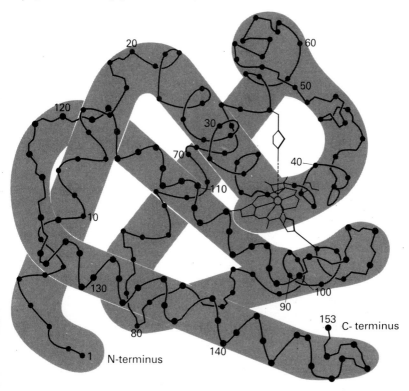

Fig. 2–5 An outline of the myoglobin molecule, indicating the polypeptide backbone. Numbers represent amino acids, with 1 starting at the N-terminal position. (Redrawn with permission from R. E. Dickerson and courtesy of Academic Press.)

Tertiary structure. We can usefully think of globin in its secondary structure as a rather stiff hollow tube. Now some proteins do utilize polypeptide chains more or less in that form, especially contractible and fibrous proteins. But for the most part proteins are roughly globular in shape, and the globins are certainly globular proteins. In order to attain a globular form, the basic α helix is closely coiled rather after the manner of a piece of elastic rubber band which has folded up on itself. The form taken by the folded coil is absolutely precise (see Fig. 2–5), and is stabilized partly by the actual preferential bending of the α helix (proline residues are particularly apt to cause local bends in the coil) but also bonding between adjacent folded sections of the helix. It is this three-dimensional tertiary structure which gives to most proteins their activity as enzymes or structural molecules—if they lose it they cannot recover it again, but are then analogous to a melted down key—the material is all there but it has lost the structure on which its significance depended. Such loss of tertiary structure in proteins is known as denaturation. Your breakfast egg, after boiling, has a firm palatable white layer of protein which has been irreversibly denatured by heating. If you can find out how to renature the white of your boiled egg, there is a Nobel Prize awaiting you!

We might ask how globin, or any other protein, acquires its unique tertiary structure. The answer seems to be not that it was moulded on a jig, but that when the amino acids are added one at a time during synthesis, the polypeptide α helix naturally coils up on itself and so acquires the special stable tertiary structure. Once lost, only resynthesis one amino acid at a time could restore the conformation.

Quaternary structure. Some proteins possess a further level of complexity in their architecture and this is referred to as quaternary structure. It describes the organization in which a number of different polypeptide chains are conjugated together to form a complex molecule. The component chains may be similar or dissimilar. For example myoglobin has no quaternary structure, since the active molecule contains only one polypeptide chain. But haemoglobin normally exists as a tetramer of four monomers, and this tetrameric organization is referred to as quaternary structure. Many other proteins such as lactic dehydrogenase also possess this fourth dimension to their final form. Each monomer in haemoglobin consists of a single globin in which one haem group is embedded, and the four monomers are held together by hydrophobic links between the adjacent polypeptide chains. These links appear to play a vital role in the physiological allostery displayed by the molecular complex (see Chapter 1). Thus, when one of the haem groups in the tetramer accepts an oxygen molecule, the globin chain in which it is lodged undergoes a small accommodating change in shape. This alteration is passed on to the other globins in the complex, so that they too undergo slight changes in tertiary structure. By doing so they alter the potential oxygen affinity of their haem groups. So the allosteric shifts of haemoglobin involve changes in both directions—an oxygen-carrying haem can alter the conformation of its associated globin, and a small change in the shape of the globin moiety can alter the oxygen affinity of the associated haem group. By a clever exploitation of these abilities, the complex molecule functions admirably as a respiratory pigment.

We should not forget, of course, that not all the subunits in haemoglobin are identical. Actually, tetramers of four like globin chains can be formed in the test tube, and occasionally occur in nature. Such homotetramers display hyperbolic oxygen saturation curves similar in shape to those given by haemoglobin monomers or myoglobin, so it is obvious that the intriguing allosteric qualities of the tetramer depend on the interactions of adjacent differing globins. Fig. 2–6 illustrates the manner in which the four monomers fit together to form the tetramer.

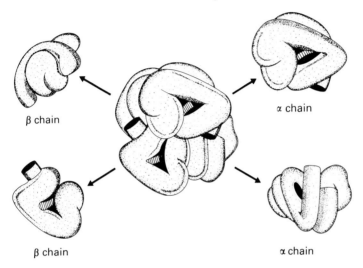

β chain

α chain

β chain

α chain

Fig. 2–6 A schematic, 'exploded' diagram showing the structure of the most common adult vertebrate Hb. Each Hb molecule contains four polypeptide chains and four haem units. (Redrawn with permission from Hochacka and Somero (1973) and courtesy of W. B. Saunders Co.)

2.3   Variations in the structure of haemoglobin

One of the most interesting aspects of haemoglobin biology is the variation in the types of haemoglobin found in different organisms and, especially at different developmental stages, within one organism. I should emphasize that when the term haemoglobin is used, it refers to the complete tetramer; when single chains are discussed they are designated as globins or monomers. Before we proceed to compare the haemoglobins and globins of different organisms, let us discuss the different haemoglobins within one organism. It is both interesting and useful to take a first look at the human haemoglobin picture.

Human haemoglobins fall neatly into three categories, each related to a particular stage of development. These three groups of molecules are referred to as embryonic, fetal, and adult haemoglobins. For the first three months of embryonic life, up to three different embryonic haemoglobins are to be found in the embryo: one of these is sometimes referred to as Portland haemoglobin, the other two as Gower haemoglobins. From two months to birth, the embryonic haemoglobins are replaced by a single type of fetal haemoglobin, and after birth the fetal type gives way to two adult types A_1, and A_2, of which A_1 (normally styled simply HbA) accounts for a rather constant 97.5% of the total haemoglobin. So we see that six different types of haemoglobin occur in normal human life. Numerous other variant forms occur, some associated with particular diseases. Two of these, haemoglobin H and haemoglobin Barts, have interesting molecular compositions which will be picked up in our discussion in a moment.

But let us turn first to the question of which globins occur in which haemoglobin. As Table 1 illustrates, human haemoglobins are chiefly

Table 1   Human haemoglobins and their subunits

Haemoglobins	Symbols	Globin subunits
Embryonic haemoglobins	HbE_1	$\alpha_2 \epsilon_2$ (Gower 2)
	HbE_2	$e_2 \zeta_2$ (Gower 1)
	HbE_3	$\zeta_2 \gamma_2$ (Portland)
Fetal haemoglobin	HbF*	$\alpha_2 \gamma_2$
Adult haemoglobins	HbA	$\alpha_2 \beta_2$
	HbA_2	$\alpha_2 \delta_2$

* *Note* The human γ chain gene is duplicated and the two copies are not absolutely identical. There are, therefore, two types of human HbF, differing in the amino acid at the 136 position.

composed of aggregates of two identical dimers, but each dimer consists of different monomers. In some cases, even in normal health, homotetramers occur and one of the embryonic haemoglobins, made up of four ϵ chains, in such a molecule. Similarly haemoglobin H occurs in some blood diseases and is a tetramer of four β chains, while haemoglobin Barts is an abnormal fetal type consisting of four γ chains. But many globins are shared by different haemoglobins, haemoglobin α sharing in HbF the fetal haemoglobin, and both adult type molecules HbA and HbA_2. So (see Fig. 2–7), birth involves a major cut down in the production of the γ globin found in the fetal tetramer, and a dramatic switch over to the synthesis of the β globin found in HbA. Table 1 reveals that six different globins are produced in a healthy human during life, and these globins are utilized to form six different haemoglobin tetramers.

That then is the human haemoglobin complement, a not uncomplicated pattern. We can now proceed to ask how the human situation

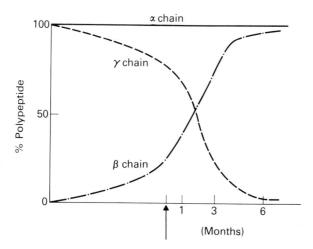

Fig. 2–7 Diagram of the changes with age in α, β, and γ chain production in the human fetus and infant. The arrow marks the birth. (From Ingram, V. M. *Haemoglobins in Genetics and Evolution.* Columbia Univ. Press, 1963.)

compares with that found in other organisms. The short answer is that the pattern is highly variable, and while most species examined do indeed have more than one type of haemoglobin, the number varies between species both during development and in adult life. The picture is clearest in the vertebrates, but still very variable. Larval fish very frequently have haemoglobins which differ from the adult, while the adults may have from two to twenty-two different haemoglobin types (the high number quoted is from the American Coho salmon). Primitive fish such as lampreys and hag fishes have either a single monomer haemoglobin or a dimer consisting of two identical monomers. There is very little information on whether different types of haemoglobin occur together in organisms below the vertebrates, but it is probably an infrequent occurrence. Amongst the vertebrates, from fishes through to man, the general architecture of the haemoglobin types is broadly similar, the molecule being a tetramer with two different kinds of subunit and an overall molecular weight of close to 68 000.

Amphibian larvae or tadpoles normally have a pattern of haemoglobin which changes during metamorphosis to the adult. For example the African clawed toad *Xenopus laevis*, which I have myself worked on for some years, has four different tadpole haemoglobins and two adult ones, one of the molecular species being common to both situations but much stronger in the adult. We have been interested in my laboratory in how the switch of haemoglobin pattern is related to amphibian metamorphosis. We have found, for example, that in the axolotl *Ambystoma*, an American salamander, the neotenous adult forms possess adult-type haemoglobin (a neotenous animal becomes sexually mature while still otherwise juvenile). On the other hand *Xenopus* tadpoles whose development is retarded by a thyroid antagonist become giant in size but larval in form. The haemoglobin of most of these 'giant' tadpoles is adult in type. Perhaps our most interesting discovery is that very anaemic adult *Xenopus* synthesize some tadpole-type haemoglobin.

Birds also show a developmental transition of haemoglobin pattern between embryo and adult. While in some species the change consists only in an alteration in ratios rather than replacement of one haemoglobin by another, the domestic fowl displays strikingly different patterns of embryonic and adult haemoglobin. These differing haemoglobin patterns seem to be correlated strongly with the site in which the blood cells themselves develop, the embryonic erythrocytes being produced by the embryonic yolk sac and the later erythrocytes from the liver. We will return in Chapter 5 to a discussion of the interesting relationship between the 'type' of erythrocyte and the 'type' of haemoglobin which it contains. The straight transition from embryonic to adult-type haemoglobins also occurs in many mammals such as the mouse and the rat, there being no intermediate group of fetal haemoglobins.

Following on this brief survey of vertebrate haemoglobins, a few points need to be stressed. The first is that in very few of these situations have the globins themselves been analysed. Clearly, with a situation which involves a very large number of haemoglobin types, the number of different globins is likely to be much smaller. If we permit homopolymers to count (tetramers of four identical globin chains) then four different globins can give rise to ten different tetramer combinations: if homopolymers are excluded the number drops to six possible tetramer combinations (assuming, of course, that each tetramer is composed of two identical dimers).

Secondly, the precise pattern sometimes varies for individuals within a species, and balanced genetic polymorphisms account for this. This interesting aspect will be discussed at greater length in Chapter 4. The metabolic state of the individual, or the prevailing environment, may also affect the pattern of haemoglobin present, ranging from production of fetal haemoglobin by anaemic adults in man, to altered haemoglobin patterns resulting from prolonged exposure to altitude in dogs.

2.4   Significance of multiple haemoglobin types

We have now come to the point where we must ask one of the most interesting and searching questions in molecular biology. That is, why does one organism have multiple types of haemoglobin? Or, more broadly, why multiple types of any other protein? We had better begin to answer that by indicating the frequency with which other proteins also occur in varied types. No doubt, next to haemoglobin, the best known example is lactate dehydrogenase (LDH) where the five types or isoenzymes of this protein consist of tetramers of two basic monomer subunits. Some other subunit types also occur but in very specialized tissues. But having cited LDH, we must pause to think of other examples. For the true situation is that for many proteins we do not know if they occur as variant types or not. If they are functionally indistinguishable and are difficult to separate by standard biochemical methods, then we remain generally ignorant about variant forms of any one protein. One must also be careful not to assume that proteins recovered in separate fractions are necessarily distinct molecular types, since changes in molecular form may occur in certain physiological conditions but do not indicate differences in primary structure. The recovery of monomers, dimers and tetramers, all composed of one monomer, is also a phenomenon which can lead to erroneous conclusions about multiple protein species. But even if these cautions are observed, one is left with the conclusion that something of the order of half of all known enzymes occur in multiple forms of slightly variant primary structure. So we can see that, in trying to find answers to the question about haemoglobin, we are facing up to a very general phenomenon in cellular protein chemistry. It is my impression that the answers which we can supply to help to explain the haemoglobin phenomenon are also generally applicable to the other protein polymorphisms as well.

There are two main answers to our question. One, in short, is that some variant forms have slightly different physiological characteristics, and so it is advantageous for the organism to possess them, providing as they do an increased fitness for the individual, especially in adapting to changing environment. We will call this the 'functional advantage' explanation. But what of differing molecules which, in the teeth of the most rigorous investigation, fail to show any variation in physiological activity? Some people argue that failure to find such variation is simply failure in the experimental approach. But others, including myself, conclude that many molecular variants exist as a result of mutation of repeated gene copies which code for that protein. They probably represent an earlier stage in molecular evolution, since variant primary structure must clearly be the background material from which evolution can select the most desirable molecular forms. We will call this the 'multiple gene copy without functional advantage' explanation. Of course it should be noted that all molecules in the 'functional advantage' category will also be coded for by multiple gene copies, and that in the course of natural selection a particular haemoglobin type might move from the category of 'no functional advantage' to the first category either by incorporating additional changes in amino acid sequence or proving fortuitously useful in a new environmental situation.

We have here begun to cover ground that is more appropriate to Chapter 4 but we will conclude this chapter by citing biological situations which demonstrate each category. The first is the possession by migratory fish such as eel and salmon of haemoglobins with very different Bohr effects. It seems plausible that these differences are functionally related to the migratory habits of these fish, some haemoglobins being optimally effective in salt water and others in fresh water. It was at one time assumed that the possession of embryonic or fetal haemoglobin by the mammalian fetus was designed to permit oxygen transport from the adult haemoglobin across the placental barrier. It is now known, however, that at least in man, the fetal and adult haemoglobins have identical oxygen affinities when extracted, and that it is a reduced affinity for intracellular diphosphoglycerate concentration of the fetal haemoglobin which serves to increase the apparent oxygen affinity of the fetal haemoglobin in the fetal erythrocyte.

Examples of the second situation are relatively frequent, ranging from the two haemoglobins A and A_2 in man, to multiple haemoglobins with identical properties in many fish. All these seem to be situations where the diverse molecules have, as yet, no functional significance and confer no adaptive advantage, only a potential for one.

3 Haemoglobin Synthesis and its Control

There is no molecule better suited than haemoglobin to act as a model for studies on protein synthesis. Its structure, size, and even its colour have made it the favoured molecular subject for such work and many classic experiments in the field of protein synthesis involve haemoglobin.

3.1 Sites of synthesis

Like many biological molecules, haemoglobin is not necessarily made in the cells in which it is most commonly found. Thus, although it is found in greatest abundance in the mature red corpuscles or erythrocytes, in most animals it is not actively made in these cells. It is in the precursors of the erythrocytes, the erythroblasts and reticulocytes, that haemoglobin synthesis is most active, and in these cells it accounts for a large proportion of the total protein manufactured.

Since haemoglobin is made up of two separate types of molecule, we will deal with each separately and then discuss how they are brought together and bonded to make the final composite structure.

3.2 Haem synthesis

As we have discussed in Chapter 2, haem is a porphyrin molecule associated with a ferrous iron atom. Our understanding of its synthesis begins with the findings of Shemin and Rittenberg that glycine (labelled with a radioactive isotope so that it could be followed) when fed to man, was found later to be incorporated into the haem of early erythrocytes. Actually what happens is that glycine is activated by association with pyridoxal phosphate, and then combines with succinate, which has been in turn activated by association with coenzyme A. The activated glycine and succinate combine, under the influence of an enzyme called δ-aminolevulinic acid synthetase, to form δ-aminolevulinic acid (ALA). Following this step, two ALA molecules are combined to form the monopyrrole porphobilinogen (PBG) and four PBG molecules are assembled together to form the large ring-shaped uroporphyrinogen. Following some modification of this ring molecule involving mainly the clipping of some of its projecting side chains, we arrive at the structure known as protoporphyrinogen IX. A ferrochelatase enzyme now pops a ferrous iron atom into the centre of the ring to yield the finished haem molecule. This pathway is summarized in Fig. 3-1.

Of perhaps greater fascination to the general biologist than how it is

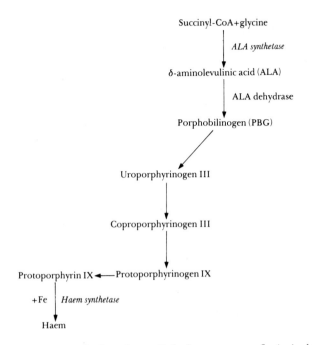

Fig. 3–1 The haem synthetic pathway. Only those enzymes of principal interest are included. The enzymes in italics are found in the mitochondria while the other enzymes are in the soluble supernatant fraction.

made is where haem is produced. Interestingly, some steps of the synthesis occur in the cellular mitochondria and others in the cytoplasm. It appears that ALA is produced in mitochondria but is then discharged into the cytoplasm for the processing which goes as far as coproporphyrinogen (an intermediate between uroporphyrinogen and protoporphyrinogen). The coproporphyrinogen then returns 'home' to the mitochondrion for further processing and insertion of the iron to yield haem. Since aerobic bacteria have the ability to synthesize haem, we can postulate that in the course of evolution, early intracellular symbiotic bacteria were originally solely responsible for haem production. With time, however, some of the steps of haem synthesis were adopted by the parent cell, and now the mitochondria, presumptive relatives of the early symbiotic bacteria, are responsible for the first and last stages of haem manufacture only.

It is also fascinating to remember that the other pigment of overwhelming importance in nature, chlorophyll, is manufactured by cells in a very similar way. Perhaps both chlorophyll and haemoglobin only became available to cells following a relationship between simple primitive cells and prokaryotes such as bacteria and blue green algae.

3.3   Globin synthesis

Globin synthesis begins at the level of the gene, for it is at that level that the primary decision is made about whether or not a particular cell should manufacture haemoglobin. To the best of our present knowledge, cells which do not make haemoglobin keep their globin genes completely silent and unexpressed. If we follow the fate of a maturing vertebrate erythroblast, then a time arrives in its development when the globin genes are first activated. We do not know how exactly this happens, although present evidence suggests that the block of DNA containing the appropriate genes is opened out from its previously condensed state, and that possibly other regulatory proteins are involved in engineering the actual switching on of the globin genes. This level of control over gene expression and protein synthesis is broadly referred to as *transcriptional control*, that is, control at the level of *transcription* of the DNA into RNA. This is termed transcription since the genetic code is not thereby altered, but simply copied into a complementary form. The later step, when the RNA copy is used to dictate the structure of the appropriate protein, involves a complete change of one code—the triplets of nucleic acid bases—into another, the amino acids of the protein. Since a change of 'language' is involved this step is referred to as *translation*.

There are no doubt many aspects to transcriptional control of globin production, only some of which we can touch on here. The enzyme which makes the appropriate RNA by copying the DNA base sequence is RNA polymerase, and clearly availability of this enzyme is a primary requirement for transcription to occur. The enzyme must also start at the correct bit of the gene, not just anywhere along its length. This crucial step, termed initiation, is known to involve a special region of the gene, the promoter region. It is the job of the promoter region to bind the RNA polymerase molecule and guide it onto the 'track' at the initiation site of the gene.

Once the polymerase molecule begins to traverse the polynucleotide chain of the DNA, it catalyses the assembly of the appropriate ribosyl nucleotides to form the growing chain of RNA. But we have skated over the question of how the polymerase enzyme knows which DNA strand to read. After all, DNA is a double helix of two complementary strands. For any one gene locus, only one of the two strands is a sense strand, the complementary strand being a nonsense strand. Lack of transcription of the nonsense strand is achieved by having the promoter gene only on the sense strand. The complement of a promoter does not itself promote. The fact that one strand of the double helix is the sense strand for one gene must not be taken to imply that it is the sense strand for all the genes on the DNA molecule. There is some evidence that each strand possesses at least some genes, but, of course, the nonsense sequence, complementary to a gene, will never itself code for a gene.

To return to our polymerase molecule traversing the length of a globin gene, what is the nature of the RNA product? The key product of the globin gene is a globin messenger RNA (mRNA) molecule, that is a species of RNA, complementary to the globin gene and able to convey that coding sequence to the cytoplasm for translation into the polypeptide chain of globin. But for many eukaryotic genes, and probably for the globin genes in particular, the primary product of transcription is an RNA molecule very much greater in size than simple globin messenger. Globin messenger RNA is known to have a sedimentation velocity of about 9S (Svedberg units, which express the speed of sedimentation), but if RNA is extracted from erythroblast nuclei, the globin message is found to be associated with a fraction of RNA of above 20S. This, the high molecular weight heterogeneous RNA, appears to be a precurser of messenger RNA, and to be processed within the nucleus to yield the final message.

Part of the processing of this high molecular weight RNA involves the attachment of some 200 adenine residues to its 3' end after initial transcription, and this tail of poly A remains attached to the final messenger RNA. What now leaves the nucleus as the carrier of the sequence information for globin is this messenger RNA with the poly A sequences but without the greater part of the high molecular weight nuclear RNA molecule. Most of that molecule has been degraded and left behind in the nucleus.

It is likely that in most cases globin messenger RNA quickly becomes associated with cytoplasmic ribosomes after it leaves the nucleus. But certainly many types of cells have mechanisms for storing some messenger RNA in an inactive form, so inserting a time lapse between gene transcription and gene expression as a protein product. The early erythroid cells of most vertebrates retain a fairly extensive endoplasmic reticulum, and so initially the ribosomes associating with the globin messenger RNA will be bound to the membranous surface. As the erythroblast matures, however, most of the endoplasmic reticulum is lost, and much of the globin synthesis proceeds on small clusters of essentially free ribosomes. Such clusters, when associated with a messenger RNA molecule, are known as polysomes (see Fig. 3–2).

We might well ask whether globin messenger RNA will associate with any ribosome, or whether there is some ribosomal specificity for particular messages. There is indeed some slight evidence in favour of ribosomal specificity in some rather special situations, but probably it is an exceptional rather than normal situation. Some ambiguity also continues to surround the precise role of the endoplasmic reticulum in protein synthesis, and just how the messenger RNA/ribosome complex involves the reticulum. Certainly the simple polysome model fails to take account of the fact that in many erythroid cells the ribosomes are bound to the reticular surface, so that the entire membranous surface is regularly studded with ribosomes.

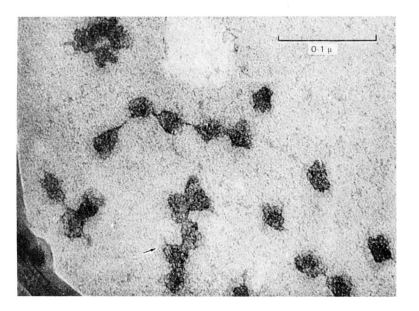

Fig. 3–2 Polyribosomes. An electron micrograph of an extract from rabbit reticulocytes showing ribosomes attached in groups to presumptive messenger RNA molecules. (Reproduced by courtesy of Dr. A. Rich.)

Once the globin messenger RNA molecule (which may sometimes be complexed to some protein to form a ribonucleoprotein conjugate) is associated with ribosomes, protein synthesis proper commences, and translation of the nucleic acid code into protein ensues. Such translation of one code into another is now known to involve matching of three nucleotide bases (on the RNA) to one amino acid (on the protein), so that a growing string of amino acids constituting the new polypeptide chain of protein is assembled at the dictate of the base sequence on the messenger RNA. Actually, the translational step is quite complicated and requires many enzymes for its execution. Most of these we will not discuss but we must not fail to mention how the individual amino acids find their way to the appropriate slot in the growing polypeptide chain. This process, perhaps the most crucial one in the entire synthetic assembly line, involves a special type of carrier molecule termed transfer RNA. A separate species of transfer RNA exists for each type of amino acid—there are just over twenty amino acids commonly found in nature—and each transfer RNA (tRNA) molecule begins its function by complexing with its appropriate amino acid somewhere in the cytoplasm. We can usefully imagine the amino acid attached to one end of the transfer RNA, and this complex now moves to a polysome where a different part of the tRNA binds to the specific triplet of bases on the messenger RNA, dictated by its own molecular specificity. So it is the transfer RNA molecule, a clover leafed structure of some 80 nucleotides in length, which has the crucial task of assembling the building blocks of protein, the amino acids, in a particular sequence dictated by the base sequence message of the RNA. At least one of the roles of the ribosome itself seems to be the stabilization of the transfer RNA molecule so that it can position its passenger, the amino acid, not only opposite the correct triplet of bases on the mRNA, but also in line with the other assembled amino acids brought by other transfer RNA molecules. As the amino acids are held in place by the tRNAs, enzymes catalyse peptide linkages between them which result in the formation of a polypeptide chain (see Fig. 3–3.)

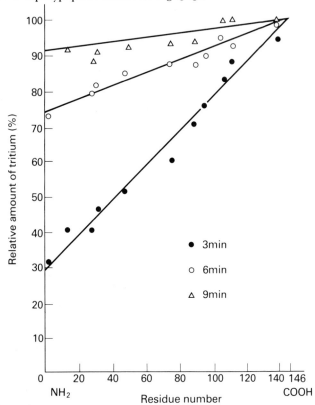

Fig. 3–3   Translation time of human β globin. Human reticulocytes were incubated with tritiated leucine for 3, 6 and 9 minutes. After incubation, chains were fingerprinted and the radioactivity of each peptide determined. Whereas at 3 minutes incubation there is wide disparity between the radioactivity of peptides at different ends of the chain, by 9 minutes all peptides are almost uniformly labelled. (From Weatherall, D. J. and Clegg, J. B. *The Thalassaemia Syndromes.* Blackwell, 1972.)

Most mRNAs are monocistronic, that is they contain the code for only one gene. Those carrying codes for a series of adjacent genes are termed polycistronic. Globin mRNA appears to be normally monocistronic and its length is only slightly greater than the 435 bases needed to code for globin, which has, on average, about 140 amino acids. When amino acids have been assembled and polymerized at the dictates of the globin mRNA, the completed globin dissociates from the polysome, or is at least free to do so when removed by yet other control factors.

We have so far talked as if a globin molecule consisted simply of a straight string of amino acids arranged in a special order. But in fact all proteins have intricate three-dimensional structures and indeed their structural or catalytic functions normally depend entirely on their three-dimensional form. How is their final architectural form engineered? The general answer is that their final structure is the most stable configuration for that particular sequence of amino acids. As the polypeptide chain grows in length, it twists and curls in order to permit stable bonding between its constituent amino acids and so the final product is a chain intricately and precisely folded upon itself in a unique way. Since this folding process can only be accomplished during assembly, any later loss of three-dimensional structure—so called denaturation—is normally irreversible and the protein can never regain its original form or function.

3.4   Haemoglobin assembly

Our discussion so far has yielded globin molecules, intricately folded to provide this unique architectural form, still sitting on the cytoplasmic polysomes of an erythroblast or reticulocyte. Taking normal human adult haemoglobin as an example, consisting as it does of two α globins and two β globins forming a tetramer, we can proceed to ask how the tetramer is assembled? The answer seems to be that the α globin chains are released from the polysomes spontaneously, or perhaps depending on the existing demand for α chains. On the other hand, some β chains seem to remain bound to the polysomes until a free α globin attaches to them and thus engineers their release. This implies that the release of β chains in the cytoplasm is partly affected by the supply of free α chains although some β chains also seem to be spontaneously released. The $\alpha\beta$ dimers which are now free in the cytoplasmic milieu, proceed to combine with the haem molecules released from the mitochondria. Haem does have some influence on the actual rate of globin synthesis on the ribosomes, but there is still doubt whether this effect is actually specific for globin rather than a generalized effect of haem on protein synthesis. Once each monomer in the $\alpha\beta$ dimer has accepted a haem group, the haemoglobin dimers conjugate spontaneously to form tetramers consisting of two α and two β chains each, the final stable and active form of adult haemoglobin.

Availability of haem also effects the size of the haemoglobin 'stockpile', and as we discussed earlier in this chapter, this is assembled from the precursor aminolevulinic acid produced by the action of the enzyme ALA synthetase. The availability and activity of this enzyme therefore exerts a very powerful influence on the rate of haem and haemoglobin production.

3.5   Haemoglobin degradation

Although, in cell biology, there is always more emphasis placed on synthesis than on degradation, it is important to grasp that the latter is often a highly important metabolic activity. Of course the blood cells themselves have a limited lifespan, the adult human erythrocyte persisting for some 120 days in circulation, and this obviously imposes a need for a constant supply of new erythrocytes. But less obvious is the controlled degradation of protein within the cell, which exerts a demand for synthesis of replacement molecules. Actually haemoglobin is probably unusual in having a very slow rate of intracellular breakdown, but none the less the mature erythrocyte at the end of its useful life has *less* haemoglobin within it than does the more active immature erythrocyte. It should be appreciated, moreover, that in the case of many proteins, very active intracellular degradation occurs, and half lives of protein survival may be measured in days or even hours.

3.6   Erythropoietin [see also section 5.3]

This substance is a glycoprotein hormone, manufactured chiefly in the kidney. Unfortunately it has not, to date, been highly purified, and preparations which demonstrate erythropoietin activity are still slightly heterogeneous. It has multiple effects on blood cell production, and protein synthesis within the blood cells. In the presence of erythropoietin the rate of maturation and release of blood cells by the erythropoietic organs is increased. In this regard the hormonal activity is complicated by the probable action of erythrocyte chalone, a substance or group of substances, released by the blood cells, which affects the rate of their own production by feed-back inhibition. We would thus suppose that, in sudden anaemia following traumatic blood loss, the kidneys would produce more erythropoietin and so stimulate increased blood cell production and release, while the level of erythrocyte chalone would fall due to the diminished total blood cell population. This reduced chalone level would also be instrumental in inducing more rapid erythropoiesis.

But of more relevance to this present chapter is the effect of erythropoietin on haemoglobin synthesis. Research on this topic is still at an early stage, and results are somewhat contradictory and confusing, but we can say that, although direct effects of the hormone on globin production are arguable, in at least some animals the hormone does stimulate haem synthesis within the immature blood cells, and, as we have seen, this is likely to affect the overall rate of haemoglobin production in turn.

4 The Genetics and Evolution of Haemoglobin

The study of haemoglobin provides an excellent insight into basic principles of genetics. Moreover, as we shall see in this chapter, some diseases which involve abnormal haemoglobin production also illuminate important molecular aspects of gene activity.

4.1 The globin genes, their detection and location

Almost all organisms above the bacteria, that is those possessing discrete nuclei, are diploid. This implies that for most of their life cycle most of the cells of these organisms possess two copies of the complete genome, and therefore two copies of each gene in that genome. The most obvious exceptions are, of course, the egg and sperm cells which are haploid (that is, they possess only one copy of each gene) and some tissue cells which are polyploid. For any one gene, the two copies may be identical or non-identical. If identical, the organism is said to be homozygous for that gene; if non-identical, heterozygous for that gene. Non-identical copies of the same gene are known as alleles or allelomorphs. Let us also pause to remind ourselves what, in molecular terms, we mean by a gene, whether it codes for globin or any other protein. A gene is basically a double helical length of DNA whose sequence of nucleotides serves as a code for the amino acid sequence of a polypeptide chain. But clearly only one of the two strands actually carries the code. As discussed in Chapter 3, the opposite strand to the sense coding strand is not transcribed, and is referred to as the nonsense strand. It is the short promoter sequence at the start of the sense strand which instructs and enables the RNA polymerase molecule to begin the read-out or transcription of the gene and the complement of a promoter does not itself promote.

We know that the DNA of higher organisms is organized into chromatin and, during cell division at least, into distinct chromosomes. We can therefore proceed to ask how many copies of each globin gene occur in an individual organism, and where on the chromosomes these genes are to be found. The only organism for which this information is available in any depth is man himself, although studies on globin gene number have also been carried out on animals such as ducks and rabbits.

In man, then, present evidence strongly suggests that there is in each haploid genome, only one gene for β globin and one for δ globin, more than one and probably two or three for γ globin, and between two and three copies of the α globin genes. This means that in most cells, and in particular within the erythrocytes, double these quoted numbers will exist, since the cells are diploid. Some ambiguity surrounds all of these figures, since it is not easy to determine the precise gene number, and the techniques involved often yield conflicting results.

It is interesting to take a brief look at the methods which have been used to ascertain the numbers of these genes. The most important is nucleic acid hybridization. This interesting but complex technique involves the isolation of globin messenger RNA from reticulocytes. Following isolation of the globin mRNA, DNA copies are synthesized in the test-tube using the mRNA as template. This process, the synthesis of DNA from an RNA template, is known as reverse transcription, and is only rendered possible by the use of a remarkable reverse transcriptase enzyme which is possessed by some tumour viruses. The nucleotides provided for the DNA synthesis in the test-tube are radioactive, so what is obtained is a preparation of globin genes which is very highly radioactive.

Total DNA is now prepared from some suitable tissue of the animal species under investigation, mixed under carefully controlled conditions with the radioactive globin DNA, and, by measuring the trapping of the radioactive DNA by the total DNA, estimates can be made of the number of genes involved in the trapping process.

A related technique to test-tube hybridization of nucleic acids is known as 'in situ' hybridization. In this approach, either radioactive globin mRNA or radioactive globin DNA, prepared as previously described, is hybridized to the DNA of cells which have been fixed on a microscope slide.

The other technique which has yielded useful information on globin gene number is that of the analysis of families with mutations at one of the haemoglobin loci. This involves the examination of individual people with abnormal haemoglobins, determining which globins are affected and whether all of that particular globin is aberrant. Moreover, in some families of affected individuals, the globin genes are found to be 'linked' to other genes, either those of other globins or other known proteins. Linked genes are those which are close together on the same chromosome and which therefore fail to show independent assortment at meiotic division. Such data can provide additional information on gene position.

Taking these techniques together, it has been possible to arrive at the numbers of genes for each globin with reasonable certainty, as well as to determine their relationship to each other. The best evidence about the numbers of α genes stems from some interesting observations on a Hungarian family with two different aberrant α chain globins, styled haemoglobin Buda and haemoglobin Pest (Budapest being the Hungarian capital). One member of this intriguing family was found to possess 25% α chain Buda, 25% α chain Pest, and 50% normal α chain. Remembering that blood cells are diploid and possess two copies of each chromosome, the simplest conclusion which would account for this situation is that the individual was heterozygous for each of two α globin genes, having one Buda globin gene, one Pest globin gene and two normal α globin genes in the diploid set—implying that at least two α globin genes occur per haploid genome, and at least four in the diploid. Curiously there is some evidence which suggests that some individuals of Oriental races possess only one α globin gene per haploid set.

In talking of homozygosity and heterozygosity we have made an assumption that deserves a little more comment. The assumption is that both copies of a single gene present in a diploid cell are equally expressed. There seems little doubt that in most cases, and particularly in relation to the genes for globin, this is correct. But it may not be invariably the case. Quite aside from the phenomenon of dominance, where the overt expression of one allelic form of a gene takes precedence over the other allele present, there are examples known where only one of two alleles present in a diploid cell is actually transcribed into RNA.

So much for gene number. We have already observed that the techniques described can actually provide information about gene position, that is the gene locus on a particular chromosome. Here again the conclusions must be slightly tentative and some assume that the human situation will be as in the mouse. They are that only two out of the 23 chromosomes in the human haploid set possess globin genes, and they are probably the large chromosomes 4 and 16. The α globin genes appear to be clustered on the long arm of chromosome 16, while all the genes for the β, γ, and δ globins are clustered on the long arm of chromosome 4. As we shall discuss later in this chapter, the adjacent positions of the last three globin genes is particularly interesting from the viewpoint of molecular and genic evolution, while the distant position of the α globin genes correlates strikingly with the distinction in primary structure of the α globin sequences.

4.2   Multiple gene copies and genic evolution

As I have just outlined, the genes for globin are multiple in two separate senses. Firstly there are separate genes coding for the different types of globin, and secondly there are at least a few separate gene copies for some of the individual globins. How and why do these multiple copies exist? This question really reaches back to the more fundamental and searching question of why organic evolution has happened in the way that it has, from small amounts of DNA to large? For, although there are curiosities in the animal and plant world which possess extravagantly great amounts of DNA, by and large the size of the total genome increases progressively with evolutionary complexity and terrestrial history. There are many interesting theories which attempt to explain the direction of evolution, and we cannot here afford space to discuss them. But what we can do is to attempt to answer the simple question of how the genome might itself increase in size. It is not difficult to conceive of ways in which this could come about. The simplest possible mechanism is probably a mistake during DNA replication, during which the DNA polymerase molecule traverses the same gene twice. A similar result might even stem from an accidental replication during gene transcription, so that a gene was replicated instead of transcribed (as is now known, both processes begin by transcription of the DNA to provide a small section of RNA primer). Other suggested mechanisms involve an unequal exchange of DNA during the process of crossing-over at meiosis.

It is, therefore, not difficult to see that, with time, multiple and identical copies of a gene might arise, normally located together on the chromosome. The next point to discuss is that such multiple copies, initially occupying adjacent loci on the chromosome, may tend to drift apart on the chromosome or genome. After all, we know of no particular reason why similar genes should be situated together, at least in terms of their transcriptional or replicative efficiency. How might genes, which began life together, drift apart in the genome? Such translocation is also most easily accounted for by unequal crossing-over at meiosis. It is well known that whole sections of chromosomes may be moved from one chromosome and become attached to another during this process. For example in the study of Down's syndrome (mongolism) it has been observed that there is an extra chromosome number 21. Normally this extra 21 is free and leads to a chromosome number of 47, with three 21 chromosomes (trisomy 21). More rarely, Down's syndrome patients have no extra full chromosome, but a much enlarged chromosome 14: clearly what has occurred is that the extra chromosome 21 has become permanently attached to one arm of chromosome 14. More commonly, translocation would involve exchange between chromosomes, so that no gene loss or increase occurred and no altered genetic expression resulted. Such translocation seems to be not uncommon in the process of meiotic division.

Now in order to understand the next stage in genic evolution, we must discuss the nature of the highly important phenomenon of mutation. A mutation can be defined as a permanent change in the base sequence of a gene (see Fig. 4–1), and such changes seem to result most frequently from the effects of cosmic radiation on the DNA. However, in recent years, biologists have become aware of the key role of certain DNA repair enzymes which have rather complex functions in repairing the deleterious changes induced by cosmic rays or other mutagenic radiations or chemicals. Interestingly enough, not only do the repair enzymes profoundly affect the effective mutation rate, but they do so substantially by *mis*repairing damaged DNA. This implies that mutation rate comes to be, to a considerable extent, under cellular control, and can be varied by altering the numbers or efficiency of the repair enzymes. Let us now assume that more than one copy of a particular globin gene exist, and that

AMINO ACID IN NORMAL HAEMOGLOBIN		AMINO ACID IN MUTANT HAEMOGLOBIN	
Lysine (AAA)	⟶	Glutamic acid (GAA)	A → G
Glutamic acid (GAA)	⟶	Glutamine (CAA)	G → C
Glycine (GGU)	⟶	Aspartic acid (GAU)	G → A
Histidine (CAU)	⟶	Tyrosine (UAU)	C → U
Asparagine (AAU)	⟶	Lysine (AAA)	U → A
Glutamic acid (GAA)	⟶	Valine (GUA)	A → U
Glutamic acid (GAA)	⟶	Lysine (AAA)	G → A
Glutamic acid (GAA)	⟶	Glycine (GGA)	A → G

Fig. 4–1 Examples of known mutations in haemoglobin. (Courtesy of Dr. W. Hexter and Dr. H. Yost, Jr., and Prentice Hall Inc.)

only one copy is necessary to satisfy the transcriptional needs of the blood cells for globin mRNA. It then follows that mutations in the other copies will not be strongly opposed by evolutionary selection. Moreover, if such mutations do not affect the efficiency of the resulting globin chain, no selective pressure will be operative against mutations in any of the gene copies. It is, of course, well known that effective mutations (ones which occur and persist) are most commonly those which affect the amino acids in uncritical parts of the polypeptide chain. Clearly, looking at globin as an example, any nucleotide change which led to an altered amino acid in that part of the globin which is critically folded and positioned round the haem group, would gravely disadvantage the individual and is not likely to survive natural selection. On the other hand, changes affecting primary structure of non-critical parts of the folded globin chain are much more likely to persist. Critical parts of a protein are commonly referred to as 'active sites', and mutations at active sites are very unlikely to persist (see Fig. 4–2.)

We would therefore expect that, with time, any one gene would be liable to change its base sequence and the resultant protein its amino acid sequence, but only in parts which were not crucial to function. Of course if a mutation at an active site actually improved the efficiency of the protein, then that mutation would indeed persist, and might confer on its fortunate 'owner' an evolutionary advantage over his fellows. In a nutshell, that is probably how natural selection normally operates. But let

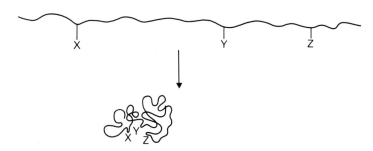

Fig. 4-2 Formation of the active site. In this diagram the polypeptide chain, containing the three amino acids whose side chains will contribute the three important binding posts of the reactive region of the enzyme (the active site), is shown at the top in an extended condition. The three reactive amino acids are at some distance from one another. At the bottom, the same polypeptide is shown in a folded configuration, which brings the three reactive side chains close together. In the folded molecule the reactive groups are brought into the proper spatial relationship to react with a particular substrate and only with that substrate. (Courtesy of Dr. W. Hexter and Dr. H. Yost, Jr., and Prentice Hall Inc.)

us return to our multiple copies of globin genes. They too will mutate, and, particularly because multiple copies exist, mutations which lead to a deviant structure in one of the resulting globins will be tolerated simply because the normal unmutated gene copy still serves the needs of the organism. So we can see that, with multiple copies, evolution can be more experimental, with the possibility that new proteins with striking new and useful properties may arise. Even if these novel molecules are of no immediate use to the organism, at some later time or place they may prove of some vital importance. It follows that possession of multiple copies with somewhat variant sequences can be a useful hedge against the unpleasant catastrophes of a changing environment. These ideas on molecular evolution were anticipated many years ago by one of the fathers of evolutionary theory, Thomas Henry Huxley. In 1869 he wrote, 'It is a probable hypothesis that what the world is to organisms in general, each organism is to the molecules of which it is composed. Multitudes of these, having diverse tendencies, are competing with one another for opportunity to exist and multiply; and the organism, as a whole, is as much a product of the molecules which are victorious as the fauna and flora of a country is the product of the victorious organic beings in it.'

On the basis of our brief résumé of evolutionary theory, we can make two predictions about globin genes. One is a recapitulation; namely that, with time, multiple copies of the same gene will move further apart. The second is that, with time, multiple copies will diverge in their sequences, and in general, the greater the divergence, the longer since the multiple copies arose. Using this sort of logic, we can look with interest at the positions and sequences of the globin genes, and sure enough they

conform to our prediction. So the genes which are most similar are also
the ones that are closest together. With these ideas in mind, the American
biochemist Vernon Ingram suggested some years ago that α was the
'ancestral' or original globin, and that probably an earlier primitive
globin gave rise to both present α globin and myoglobin. Then, as shown
in Fig. 4–3, he suggests that α gave rise to γ, γ to β and finally δ diverged
from β. The multiple copies of α and γ globin provide yet further scope
for evolutionary divergence in the future.

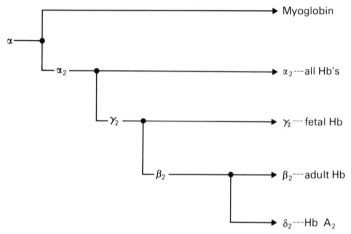

Fig. 4–3   Presumed evolution of the globin chains of haemoglobin and myo-
globin. The point in time of a gene duplication is indicated by a solid black circle.
(From Ingram, V. M. *Haemoglobins in Genetics and Evolution*. Columbia Univ.
Press, 1963.)

So far, we have talked as if all individuals within a species possessed an
identical pattern of haemoglobin at a particular developmental stage.
This is certainly untrue, for very often a population of individuals is itself
variant, and this variation may settle down to a stable pattern. Such a
phenomenon is termed balanced polymorphism. Many such
polymorphisms in nature involve the shape or colouration of the
individual, for example the pink, yellow and banded form of the common
banded snail *Cepea nemoralis*. Balanced polymorphisms also exist at the
molecular level and indeed presumably all have their basis there. So we
will not be surprised to find examples of balanced polymorphism among
haemoglobins. The haemoglobins of horses and mice are particularly
noteworthy examples where the adults within the species show variation,
and other variants exist in any population at a fixed ratio. Some minor
haemoglobin variants in man amount to balanced polymorphisms, as
indeed does sickle cell haemoglobin, in which, although the homozygote
is severely disadvantageous, the heterozygote is probably slightly

favoured. So human populations in Africa show balanced ratios of individuals with normal β globin and those with sickle cell globin. This we will discuss in greater depth in the next section.

In chapter 3 we briefly outlined the probable explanations for multiple haemoglobins, some being of obvious adaptive advantage, others offering no present benefit. We can see that what we had to say about the functional haemoglobins now marries up with what we have established about genic evolution. Some haemoglobins have come to be a potent asset to the organism possessing them, such as those with widely different Bohr effects in migratory fish. Others, such as human δ globin, seem of no particular significance to the organism, and even human γ is of less moment than is often supposed. So our multiple haemoglobins are a mixed bag, some offering biochemical advantages in special developmental or environmental situations, others being only grist for the mill of future evolution and yet others a 'hang-over' from past evolutionary history. Before we conclude this chapter we must discuss some pathologies which involve aberrant haemoglobins. These will both illustrate and extend our present discussion of the molecular evolution of the haemoglobins.

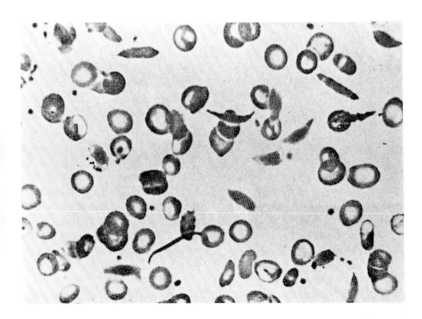

Fig. 4–4 Fresh blood from a patient with sickle cell anaemia taken during a sickling crisis. Note occasional sickle cells are present together with numerous early sickled forms. (From Lehmann, H. and Huntsman, R. G. *Man's Haemoglobins*. North Holland, 1974.)

4.3   Sickle cell anaemia

This disease is common in West and Central Africa, and also occurs in parts of India, the Persian Gulf Region, and the Central Mediterranean. Persons suffering from the disease are severely anaemic and the red blood cells which they possess are frequently of an abnormal and somewhat spiky shape, and some are distinctly sickle shaped (see Fig. 4–4). The anaemia is a direct consequence of the aberrant blood cells, since these blood cells have a reduced life span, much less than the 120 days survival of the normal human red blood cell. Red cells of patients suffering from the disease are not always mis-shapen, but they become so in conditions of low oxygen tension, which can be induced by exercise or fatigue. It appears that the irregular shape is caused by a semi-crystalline mass of haemoglobin in the cell, the protein having come out of solution at the reduced oxygen tension. The cause of the poor solubility of this haemoglobin we will discuss in a moment. Sickle cell anaemia is an extremely serious disease and is frequently fatal in the early years of life.

Besides the severe form of the disease, a related condition exists known as sickle cell trait. Individuals with sickle cell trait are not anaemic since their red blood cells have a normal life span, nor do their erythrocytes become sickle shaped under normal conditions. But if their red blood cells are exposed to very low oxygen tensions in the test-tube, they too become mis-shapen. It is now established that the two conditions of sickle cell trait and sickle cell anaemia are clearly related and genetically controlled by a single gene. Persons suffering from the disease are homozygous for the sickle cell allele while those having sickle cell trait are heterozygous, that is only one chromosome carries the 'sickle cell' form of the gene, the homologous chromosome carrying the normal form.

4.3.1   Haemoglobin S

The gene concerned in sickle cell anaemia is that coding for β globin, and in patients with the disease the β globin is of a slightly aberrant form and the resulting tetramer is termed haemoglobin S. Following on Linus Pauling's discovery of the distinct haemoglobin S, Vernon Ingram was able to demonstrate that the difference between normal β globin and sickle cell β globin is only in one amino acid—the glutamic acid in the sixth position in the β globin chain has been replaced by a valine. This alteration in one amino acid actually requires only a single base substitution in the genetic code for β globin, namely replacement of the thymine in the centre of the triplet coding for glutamic acid by an adenine to give the triplet code for valine. So we can see that the person suffering from sickle cell disease has an adenine instead of a thymine in the seventeenth nucleotide of the gene for β globin, situated, as we now know, somewhere on the long arm of each fourth chromosome. Individuals

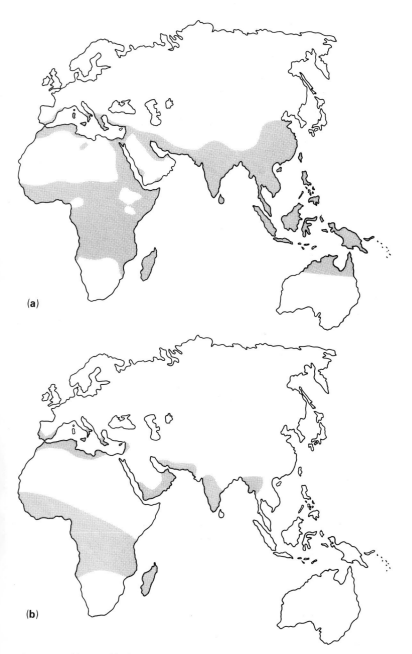

Fig. 4-5 (a) World distribution of malignant malaria. (b) Distribution of haemoglobin S in Africa. (From Lehmann, H. and Huntsman, R. G. *Man's Haemoglobins.* North Holland, 1974.)

with sickle cell trait carry this allele on only one of their two number 4 chromosomes: the other carries the normal β allele with a thymine residue in that position. The precise reason why sickle cell globin, when deoxygenated, is so insoluble, is not at present clearly understood, but it no doubt follows from a slight change in the tertiary folding of the β chain.

One of the conclusions which we can draw from these facts about sickle cell anaemia is that only one gene for β globin exists in the human haploid genome, a point which we established earlier in this chapter. We should also pause to consider the very striking clinical consequences which follow from what has presumably been a simple mutation in one gene. As Pauling has pointed out, sickle cell anaemia is truly a molecular disease. Another interesting point which emerges from studies on this fascinating disease is that, if blood from new-born infants with sickle cell disease is tested, all the erythrocytes can be induced to sickle. Yet at birth such babies have still a high level of fetal haemoglobin. It follows that both HbS and HbF must be present together in many or all of the cells—a point we will return to in Chapter 5.

4.3.2   Advantages for heterozygosity

One puzzling feature of sickle cell anaemia is its prevalence. The number of individuals with sickle cell trait and sickle cell disease seems to be much larger than one would expect for an allele which is such a severe handicap to reproduction in the homozygous condition. Now a neat explanation for its prevalence would be that the heterozygotes with sickle cell trait were not just neutral to evolutionary selection, but were actually at an advantage over the 'wild type' individual with two normal β globin alleles. This fascinating possibility was first suggested by J. B. S. Haldane and elaborated by A. C. Allison. If we take a careful look at Fig. 4–5B we will see that the disease has a very curious geographical distribution. Another common disease has a rather similar distribution, namely malaria (see Fig. 4–5A). In malaria, the protozoan parasite spends much of its life cycle inside the red blood cell. Supposing red cells of individuals with sickle cell trait made poor homes for malarial parasites! In that case the heterozygotes for sickle cell globin might be greatly advantaged as compared with normal individuals in countries with a high incidence of malaria. So there would actually be a selection *for* being a HbS heterozygote although *against* being the HbS homozygote. It has now been fairly generally accepted that this idea truly explains the prevalence of sickle cell anaemia in tropical countries.

4.4   Thalassemia

Thalassemia is really a group of diseases, all inherited, as is sickle cell anaemia, and particularly common in Central Mediterranean areas, Middle East and South East Asia. As shown in Fig. 4–6, it is particularly common in countries such as Italy (where carriers of the disease are

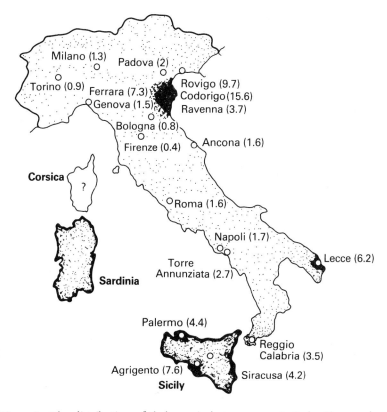

Fig. 4–6 The distribution of thalassemia heterozygotes in Italy. Figures give the percentage incidence in the various districts shown. (From Ingram, V. M. *Haemoglobins in Genetics and Evolution*. Columbia Univ. Press, 1963.)

numbered in millions), and indeed the word thalassemia stems from the Greek word 'thallos', meaning 'the sea' because it was particularly common in the Mediterranean coastal region (see Fig. 4–7). The most serious form of thalassemia is termed thalassemia major or Cooley's anaemia, and less severe forms are referred to as thalassemia minor. Patients with thalassemia, particularly thalassemia major, are anaemic, apparently because their erythrocytes are either destroyed in the marrow

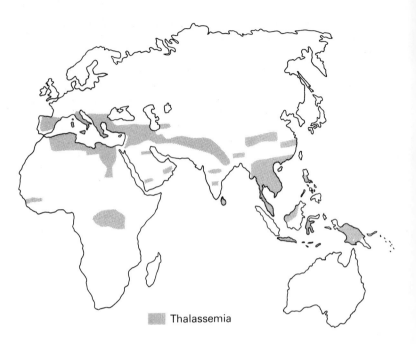

Fig. 4–7 World distribution of β thalassemia. (From Lehmann, H. and Huntsman, R. G. *Man's Haemoglobins*. North Holland, 1974.)

during maturation or recognized as aberrant and destroyed by the spleen prematurely. Although the thalassemias are a somewhat complex group of syndromes, it is reasonable to generalize by saying that thalassemia major is the homozygous condition where the aberrant allele is present in the double dose, while thalassemia minor is used to designate the heterozygous state. Thalassemia minor is often clinically symptomless. Within each of these broad genetic classes, there are many variables, the simplest being β thalassemia and α thalassemia. These terms indicate conditions in which the genetic lesion is in the β and α globin genes respectively.

Unlike sickle cell anaemia, which involves a single, clearly defined allelic form of β globin, the lesions involved in thalassemia are variable and the results often complex. For example, since α globin is present in both human adult haemoglobins and the fetal form, all these molecules will be affected by any lesion in the α chain. Moreover, since, as we have already discussed, there are multiple copies of the α globin gene, it will be possible to have some normal α globin and some abnormal.

Probably we should not overstress the point, but it is worth noting that the prevalance and geographical incidence of thalassemia provide a picture not unlike that of sickle cell anaemia. It may be that resistance to malaria can be involved as a possible factor in determining the pattern. But the theory seems less certain here than in the case of sickle cell disease.

What is of more interest to us, however, is the molecular biology of some thalassemias. Firstly, most cases of β thalassemia major are known to involve complete lack of β globin chains, and one might have predicted that this must result from a genetic deletion of the appropriate gene. However, molecular hybridization with purified α and β complementary human DNA (prepared as described earlier in this chapter) has confirmed the presence of the β globin gene in the thalassemia patients. So the lesion appears to be in a control gene which effects either the transcription of the β globin gene or processing of the β globin messenger RNA.

The completed β globin mRNA itself has proved to be absent in many affected patients. Another interesting aspect of the disease is that affected adults have a high level of fetal haemoglobin, indicating some measure of persistent γ chain synthesis as a compensation for the lack of β chains. Indeed in some individuals the synthesis of fetal haemoglobin is so extensive that compensation for the lack of adult haemoglobin A is complete. Such individuals are clinically normal and are simply said to have hereditary persistence of fetal haemoglobin. They are, however, undoubtedly more correctly seen as individuals with genetic β thalassemia in which compensation is complete. Most people affected with β thalassemia major also synthesize more δ globin and therefore have more haemoglobin A_2 (in real terms, not just proportionately more) than normal individuals. It is worth noting also that the clinical normality of adults in whom the normal haemoglobin A is replaced by haemoglobin F, serves to emphasize a point hinted at earlier—that the change from fetal to adult-type haemoglobin during mammalian development is probably more an evolutionary hang-over than a crucial physiological adaptation to the switch from a uterine to a terrestrial environment.

In contrast to β thalassemia, α thalassemia major (also known as haemoglobin Barts or hydrops fetalis) DNA is apparently lacking in α globin genes. These genes are known to be multiple, and the hybridization data cannot at present exclude the possibility that one copy of the α globin gene may persist in some cases. α thalassemia major also confirms for us the crucial importance of the haemoglobin molecule being a mixed tetramer. The disease presents in infants as a rapidly fatal condition characterized by the presence of haemoglobin Barts which is a homo-tetramer of γ chains ($γ_4$), with lesser amounts of what has come to be termed haemoglobin H, which is the β homotetramer ($β_4$). Sole possession of such haemoglobins is scarcely compatable with life and the infants are normally still-born or die within hours of birth. A disease that is normally styled 'haemoglobin H disease', is characterized by fairly mild anaemia and between 4 and 30% of the adult haemoglobin is the homotetramer β_4. This disease obviously represents an inbalance in the α to β chain ratio and is sometimes termed thalassemia intermedia.

We have only lightly skirted round the many interesting aspects of the thalassemias. While this group of diseases has already proved very illuminating in terms of molecular genetics, many intriguing questions remain unanswered. But our short discussion serves to underline the physiological importance of correct haemoglobin assembly, the strong confirmatory evidence of the thalassemia syndromes for globin gene numbers, and the interesting compensatory control of haemoglobin production in which lack of haemoglobin A may be compensated by production of A_2 and F.

5 The Red Cell

Haemoglobins are found almost exclusively inside very specialized cells, the erythroid cells, of which the mature example is the erythrocyte or red blood cell. The exceptions to this statement are discussed briefly in Chapter 1, such as the extracellular haemoglobin of some worms and the haemoglobins of yeasts and ciliates. But the relationship between haemoglobin and the red blood cell is so strong that I will devote this chapter to a discussion of the biology of these interesting cells.

5.1 Development and differentiation of the red cell

Many different cell types can be found in the blood, of which the most abundant is the erythrocyte. These cells are not normally produced in the blood, that is, they do not arise by division of pre-existing circulating blood cells. Rather they are shed into the blood from organs, the so-called erythropoietic (blood-forming) organs, and so we should first of all focus our attention on these organs, their location and function.

The blood-forming tissues are not fixed to one locality during development in any one animal, and even in adult life, more than one tissue possesses erythropoietic competence. In the earliest embryonic production of blood cells, they arise in the so-called yolk sac of the embryo, and, as the embryo forms and matures, this function is taken over by kidney, spleen, liver and lymph nodes. Finally, in adult life, the red blood cell forming tissues come to be located chiefly in the marrow of the bones, especially in vertebrae, ribs, sternum, and the long bones such as femur and humerus. But in adult life the potential for some erythropoiesis continues elsewhere and in pathological conditions such as anaemia the liver and spleen may once more become important contributors. The precise details of the changing erythropoietic sites also varies considerably in different animals, both during embryonic development and in adult life. So the kidney in fishes, the liver in amphibians and the bone marrow in mammals are the main adult sites of red blood cell production. We can also see that blood is produced by an archipelago of different sites, since even the marrow is located in many different bones, and the blood itself contributes the continual link between these sites. Primitive cells can also move readily from one of these sites to another via the blood. The changes in erythropoietic sites during the course of development of an animal, coupled with the switch from embryonic or fetal haemoglobin to adult haemoglobin pose the question of whether one erythropoietic cell line, undergoing maturation at one site, is exclusively devoted to the manufacture of one type of haemoglobin whilst another cell line synthesizes a different haemoglobin. We will delay answering this question for a little, however, until we have discussed the differentiation of the erythrocyte itself.

While it is relatively easy to recognize mature red blood cells not only by their distinctive shape, but by their being full of the red pigmented haemoglobin, the early blood cells possess little or no respiratory pigment and so their identification is much more difficult. But if we refer to Fig. 5–1, we will see that the so-called erythropoietic series involves division of a multipotential stem cell to yield the proerythroblast, which divides to yield an erythroblast. Although the erythroblasts themselves also divide, haemoglobin synthesis commences in these cells. Division of the erythroblasts yields the normoblast, which, as far as division is concerned, is the end of the line, for it is the maturation and not the division of the normoblast which finally yields the erythrocyte. Normoblasts are circular, nucleated cells with many mitochondria and a fairly extensive endoplasmic reticulum. But as they mature much of this fine structure is lost. In the mammal even the nucleus is extruded, yielding the reticulocyte, a blood cell with only the remains of the once extensive endoplasmic reticulum left in the cytoplasm. Very rapidly this remaining reticulum is destroyed, leaving essentially an empty sac of haemoglobin with a few enzymes, which constitutes the mature mammalian erythrocyte.

Differentiation of non-mammalian red blood cells is less extreme, since the nucleus is retained, although it becomes very inactive, and the mature erythrocyte remains as an oval, slightly flattened disc rather than the indented circular discus shape of the mammalian red blood cell.

One or two additional points about the production of erythroid cells are worth making. The first is that not only do lymphoid organs frequently act as sites of blood cell production, but that red blood cells and lymphocytes are probably the products of essentially the same stem cells. So the multipotential stem cell in the bone marrow of an adult man has presumably the capacity to fill three quite distinct needs—one, the need for more stem cells, i.e. self maintenance by division; another, the need for production of lymphoid cells; and thirdly, the need for production of erythroid cells. There are few better examples of tissue differentiation than this. We should note that both the mature lymphocyte and the mature erythrocyte are essentially *end* cells, incapable of division and so unable to produce more of themselves. The responsibility for continued production of these cells therefore lies with the less differentiated stem cells. We can therefore visualize the stem cells as a production unit of essentially embryonic or undifferentiated cells, continually replenishing the supply of erythroid and lymphoid cells which themselves have a strictly limited life span. Of course not all

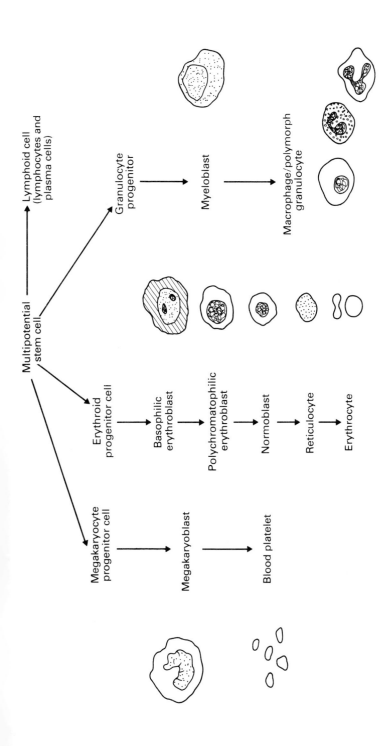

Fig. 5–1   Differentiation of the erythroid cells. Presumptive cell linkages within the human haemopoietic system.

differentiation operates in this way. In tissues such as cartilage or muscle, the functional cells themselves remain capable of division and self renewal. The other extreme is found in the neuron, which is not only incapable of division, but no stock of stem cells is retained. Neurones lost during our lifetime are never replaced and so ageing involves, and is no doubt partly a result of, the gradual reduction in the overall number of neurones.

To return to the erythroid cells, it is worth pausing to think carefully about the important steps which constitute the differentiation of the erythrocyte. The proerythroblast, for example, is a relatively 'normal' animal cell, not markedly differentiated and closely resembling many other cells found throughout the animal body. It has a large nucleus actively transcribing ribosomal and transfer RNA and a host of different types of messenger RNA. The cytoplasm around the nucleus is highly structured and elaborately compartmentalized. Numerous mito- chondria, which themselves possess DNA as their own genome, are the site of activity of the respiratory chain enzymes, and are also the production sites for various important molecules including haem. An extensive series of tubules and lamellae constitutes the membranous endoplasmic reticulum, copiously studded with ribosomes on one side. It is here that the messenger RNA molecules from the nucleus come to have their messages translated into protein. In shape the proerythroblast is more or less amoeboid, with a highly dynamic plasma membrane at the cell surface. From our point of view the fact to note is that although the cell is already fixed in its fate to become an erythrocyte (it is *determined*, in the language of embryology), it has, as yet, none of the hallmarks of the erythroid cell series.

If we now consider the late erythroblast or early normoblast we will see that many changes have ensued. The mitochondria are less numerous and are now devoted largely to the production of haem. What was once an elaborate endoplasmic reticulum is less extensive, and more of the ribosomes can be seen as free clusters, often termed polysomes. These ribosomal clusters are still highly active in protein synthesis, but are less associated with the membranous reticulum. Messenger RNA production by the nucleus is now largely confined to globin message, and transcription of other genes, including those for ribosomal and transfer RNA, is greatly reduced. In response to the direction of the nucleus via the repertoire of messenger molecules, the cytoplasmic ribosomes are now mainly dedicated to translating globin message, and haemoglobin production in all its stages accounts for the greatest part of the cell's activities.

Lastly, let us take a look at the final product in mammals, the mature erythrocyte. Here the nucleus has gone, so no more transcription can occur. The reticulum and almost all the ribosomes have gone, so virtually no translation is possible. Many other structures and molecules have also been discarded, to leave a terminally differentiated structure scarcely deserving the term 'cell'. A sac of haemoglobin, with some other proteins such as carbonic anhydrase also present, and a somewhat rigid membrane vital to retain the permeability properties of the erythrocyte. The nucleated erythrocytes of non-mammalian vertebrates, retaining a slightly active nucleus in some cases, are somewhat less extremely differentiated than the mammalian red blood cell (see Fig. 5–2). A little transcription and translation trickles on, and even the odd mitochondrion persists, but none the less the non-vertebrate erythrocyte is still to all intents and purposes a sac of haemoglobin with an inert and highly condensed nucleus in the centre.

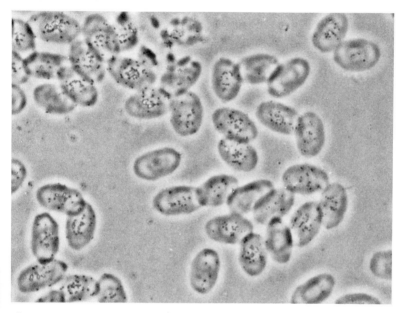

Fig. 5–2   Autoradiograph of chicken red blood cells, following culture in a medium providing tritiated uridine. The black grains are indicative of RNA synthesis.

5.2   Haemoglobin in the red cell

We can now return to the intriguing question about the correlation between the site of origin of a red cell and the type of haemoglobin which it synthesizes. We should admit immediately that the situation is a little confused and that a simple general principle does not seem to apply. Let us begin by asking the simple question of whether more than one type of haemoglobin ever coexists in the same red cell. After all, since haemoglobin is itself a mixed tetramer, we already know that more than one globin gene is expressed in each cell. The answer is in the affirmative. The minor adult haemoglobin in man, HbA_2, is found distributed throughout all the cells and not confined to a special small population. Again there is good evidence that, during human development, the fetal haemoglobin occurs in many of the same cells as the adult. This conclusion emerges clearly from new-born infants suffering from sickle cell anaemia. Electrophoresis of haemoglobin from such infants demonstrates that much fetal haemoglobin is present, yet all of their blood cells become mis-shapen (sickled) at low oxygen tensions. This implies that HbF and HbS coexist in many of the cells.

An opposite conclusion emerges, however, from observations of the distribution of fetal haemoglobin in adults, especially in pathologies such as anaemia, or hereditary persistence of fetal haemoglobin. Here the bulk of the HbF is confined to a few cells, although even in these cells a little HbA is probably also present. It is tempting and plausible to conclude that this situation arises because the cells containing HbF arise from a different erythropoietic site than those containing only adult haemoglobin, and that this site might be one normally operative only or chiefly in early development, i.e. the liver.

If we now turn to other vertebrates we can find examples of both phenomena. For example, the embryonic haemoglobins of the chick are confined to cells of yolk sac origin, while the adult chick haemoglobins occur exclusively in cells of the 'adult' series which are produced by other erythropoietic sites. Amphibians provide examples of both situations however. In some species the larval and adult haemoglobins occur in identifiably different cells which may well have different tissue origins, in other species both larval and adult haemoglobins are found together in what is apparently one line of cells. Actually it is not at all easy to unequivocally identify the types of haemoglobin inside a single red cell. The experiment is most frequently undertaken by raising separate antibodies to the differing haemoglobins in, say, rabbits, and then conjugating each antibody with a different colour of fluorescent dye. Blood cells can then be exposed to the fluorescent antibodies, smeared on a slide, and observed in an ultra-violet microscope (in which the dyes will fluoresce). Red cells fluorescing in different colours are identified as possessing the haemoglobin against which the specific antisera were raised. Any red cells containing both haemoglobins will fluoresce with both colours simultaneously.

Of course we should not be surprised, in hindsight, that some observations suggest that separate haemoglobins are confined to distinct lines of cells, while other observations confirm coexistence in the same cell. After all, organisms are physiologically extremely variable and adaptable, and much of the point of the organization of different sites of erythropoiesis in the same organism must be to permit flexibility and a modulated response to physiological stress. And, of course, even multiple erythropoietic sites are presumably only islands of tissue originally seeded from one line of cells. So we can conclude that in some situations erythroid differentiation is taken to the extreme, in which only one type of haemoglobin is synthesized in a single erythroid cell, and separate differentiated lines of erythrocytes are produced. In others, however, flexibility persists, and the globin gene expression is modulated by the environmental experience of the individual cell.

5.3   Control of red cell production [see also section 3.6]

A moment's thought will indicate that some fairly clever mechanisms must be in operation to control the cell number of any tissue. After all, during normal life the cell population of any individual tissue must at least replace cells which are lost by damage or cell death, but since tissues must remain at a fixed size the rate of cell division must not be such as to more than compensate for cell loss. When one considers the necessity of tissues also compensating for traumatic injury, where loss of skin or liver often leads to actual replacement of the missing cells, it is clear that the rate of cell production in a tissue must be very nicely controlled.

Red cell production is particularly interesting in that the differentiated cells of the erythroid tissue are not themselves capable of mitosis. This implies that the erythropoietic stem cells are the ones on which the responsibility rests for modulating supply to necessity and demand. At least two quite distinct mechanisms are commonly involved in the regulation of red cell number. The first involves the hormone erythropoietin. This substance has not been highly purified but is probably a glycoprotein, and in mammals at least, is synthesized in kidney cells. Although its effects on erythroid tissues are multiple and complex, its clearest effect is to increase production and release of red cells from the erythropoietic tissues into the circulation. In short, it induces an increase in red cell number. We have already commented that both lymphoid and erythroid cells may arise from common stem cells, and it seems possible that what erythropoietin does to the erythropoietic stem cells is not just to lead to faster mitosis, but to induce a certain type of stem cell mitosis which will specifically shed cells into the erythroid cell 'compartment'. Presumably the multipotential stem cells have the ability to divide to produce either two daughter stem cells, two daughter lymphoid cells, two daughter erythroid cells, or two cells which represent some mixture of these cell types, e.g. one stem cell plus one erythroid cell.

Test-tube studies with erythropoietin have confirmed its ability to increase the mitotic rate of the stem cells, while *in vivo* studies have demonstrated the comparative lack of species specificity displayed by the hormonal complex. Thus erythropoietin from sheep (normally isolated from the blood of sheep which have been rendered anaemic by experimental blood loss) is effective in increasing red cell production in man, and in my own laboratory we have found sheep erythropoietin to be effective in the amphibian *Xenopus*.

Now it is well known that increased red cell production in man and many other animals follows from continuing exposure to low oxygen tensions (hypoxia) such as are encountered at high altitude. So athletes or mountaineers who train at high altitudes become polycythemic (abnormally high red cell count) and so become physiologically adapted to arduous activity at high altitude. (Some animals are also reported as compensating by synthesizing haemoglobin with an increased oxygen affinity, say an embryonic or fetal haemoglobin: this phenomenon has never been recorded in man.) How then is erythroid cell production sensitive to altitude or to hypoxia, or both? It now seems certain that what is involved is sensitivity of erythropoietin production in the kidney to tissue anoxia (lack of oxygen). Increased tissue anoxia leads to increased erythropoietin production, which in turn induces production and release of greater numbers of red blood cells from the erythropoietic tissues. This sensitive relationship between oxygen tensions and red cell production operates quite rapidly, and certainly within a few hours of exposure to increased or decreased oxygen tension.

Besides the erythropoietin system, there is some evidence that a second system of regulation operates in erythroid cell production, this time involving a feed back signal from the circulating red cells to the erythropoietic tissues, so that high circulating red cell numbers automatically reduce the rate of red cell production. To date the evidence for such a system governing red cell production is somewhat slender. It rests on experiments in mice and amphibians in which sera from polycythemic individuals apparently reduces red cell production in normal or even in anaemic individuals. Such factors which regulate tissue cell production by feed back inhibition have been termed chalones, and certainly there is good evidence for the existence and operation of chalones in other tissues. They are defined as tissue specific molecules, produced by differentiated tissue cells, and having the power to retard mitosis in the same tissue. It is also likely that they are very unstable, so that sudden depletion of a tissue would be rapidly followed by reduction in the level of circulating tissue chalone, to be followed by an increase in the mitotic index of that tissue. We can conclude that there is reasonable evidence supporting the action of a chalone in erythropoiesis in some animals, but that the system is certainly less important than erythropoietin in maintaining overall control of red cell number.

In concluding our discussion of the control of red cell number, we should remember that it also depends on a regulated destruction and removal of old erythrocytes. The erythrocyte survives for approximately 120 days in human circulation. This compares with down to 25 days in some birds and up to many hundreds of days in some amphibians. What we must appreciate is that this is itself an important aspect of the regulation of red cell number. As the mature erythrocyte ages and its membrane becomes distorted, it becomes progressively more likely that in its normal passage through organs such as the spleen, it will be trapped there and broken down by phagocytes and enzymic destruction. Many anaemic conditions result not from under-production of red cells, but from their premature ageing and destruction.

5.4 The red cell surface

We will now conclude our short discussion of red cell biology by considering the remarkable properties of the red cell surface, both as regards its shape and its molecular properties. Although I have previously referred to the mature mammalian red cell as a sac of haemoglobin, that description is something of an oversimplification. For even without a nucleus and without any protein or RNA synthesis, some biochemical mechanisms persist within the structure. In particular the outer membrane retains impressive properties of controlled permeability to many molecules. The mammalian erythrocyte has also made a substantial contribution to our knowledge of cell surface membranes, since it can be broken (lysed) very easily, releasing its contents. Preparations of red cell membrane (red cell ghosts, as they are called) are one of the purest fractions of the cell membrane available to the experimenter.

The mature human erythrocyte is a biconcave flattened disc, 8.4 microns in diameter, 2.4 microns thick (a micron is $\frac{1}{1000}$th millimetre) at the periphery, and narrowing to only 1.0 micron thickness in the centre of the disc. It is composed of 71% water, 28% haemoglobin, 7% lipid such as cholesterol and lecithin, and 3% sugar, salts and other proteins. It contains about 400 million molecules of haemoglobin, accounting for 95% of its dry weight. The shape of the red cell varies with its environment, and as seen in Fig. 5–3 readily becomes spherical and crenulated if the cells are washed free of plasma. These crenulated erythrocytes are termed echinocytes, and are occasionally found in circulating blood. These shape changes are entirely reversible, and point to the fact that the normal shape is accomplished by function of elastic and skeletal properties of the cell surface. Red cells can be induced to become biconcave discs even when devoid of contents. The proteins which give the red cell surface its elastic properties may well be contractile, and one such fraction, isolated from the ghosts of human red cells, has been termed spectrin. Cross-sections of red cell membranes, when examined by electron microscopy, reveal a single unit membrane of some 70 Ångstroms thickness, but its surface is not entirely uniform, being subdivided into plaques, and the cholesterol content of the surface membrane is also obviously very high. The surface also has a fairly high net negative charge, although the magnitude of the charge diminishes with the age of the cell.

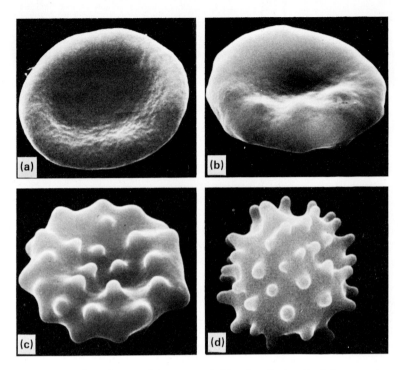

Fig. 5–3 Varying shapes of human red blood cell visualized by scanning electron microscopy. (a) is a normal biconcave red cell, sometimes referred to as a discocyte. (c) and (d) are crenulated erythrocytes with spicules, and are termed echinocytes. (b) indicates a transitional state. (Courtesy of Dr. M. Bessis and Springer-Verlag.)

The existence of molecular irregularities on the red cell surface is also verified by studies of its immunological properties. Some of the red cell surface proteins are potent antigens, and elicit powerful immunological responses in foreign organisms. These give to the blood cells their well known 'blood type' criteria of the differing blood groups. (Curiously enough, many animals, including man, carry so-called natural antigens to blood groups which they have never themselves encountered. This often implies an immediate hostile immunological response to an injection with foreign blood cells.) The blood group antigens are proteins on the red cell surface, and studies with suitable tagged antibodies reveal that these proteins are distributed patchily on the erythrocyte surface.

That the shape of the erythrocyte can be affected by its contents is, of course, demonstrated by the blood of patients suffering from sickle cell anaemia. The low solubility of their haemoglobin leads to intracellular crystals and loss of red cell shape. The biconcave disc of the mature human erythrocyte ensures that at no point in the cell is the intracellular haemoglobin far from the cell surface. When human erythrocytes become spherical they have been calculated to lose 40% of their effective surface area and become 20% less effective in terms of oxygen transport.

The erythrocyte membrane also operates as an important interface in the movement of molecules such as glucose, sodium and potassium ions, and of course water, in and out of the cell. Erythrocytes continue to utilize glucose via the pentose phosphate and Embden–Meyerhof pathways (two important pathways of carbohydrate metabolism) to provide energy for the cell. Some of this energy is also used to drive a so-called 'pump' or carrier system which governs the entry of potassium ions and exit of sodium ions against the flow of their prevailing gradients. The membrane also permits very rapid entry of small ions such as chloride and carbonate, while large molecules such as the proteins of the blood plasma are entirely excluded. All this implies that erythrocytes are highly sensitive to their osmotic environment but do retain considerable control over their internal environment. If you have a nose bleed and accidentally stain fabric with blood, we all know that a quick rinse in cold water will remove the mark, a wash in very hot water may make it permanent. This is understood easily as an effect on the red cell membrane. Cold water will enter the cells and rapidly burst or lyse them, releasing their red pigment, which can then be washed free. Very hot water will denature the proteins of the cell surfaces, binding them to the fabric and trapping the already denatured haemoglobin within. The permanent brown stain will result from the haemoglobin denaturation inside the red cells. Red cell lysis is illustrated in Fig. 5–4.

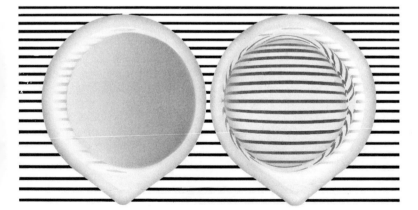

Fig. 5–4 Osmotic effects on red cells. A photograph of two beakers placed on a striped backcloth. Both contain a suspension of erythrocytes, but in the left hand vessel the cells are intact and the solution therefore opaque. The right hand vessel contains cells in water, and the water has entered the cells osmotically, followed by swelling of the cells and rupture of the membrane. This permits leakage of the haemoglobin out of the cells and a change to transparency in the solution. (Redrawn with permission of Dr. A. Solomon.)

6 Some Interesting Techniques and Experiments

Because haemoglobin is such an interesting and informative molecule it is useful to outline some of the techniques which have proved effective in studying it. Some of these methods are relatively simple and can be easily undertaken in a school science laboratory. With a few millilitres of blood, obtained painlessly from a chicken or a mouse, a host of fascinating and educative experiments are possible. References which provide details of such experimental techniques are to be found at the end of this chapter. In this chapter I will outline the most important methods which are routinely used in isolating and studying haemoglobin, and also describe some of the classic experiments which have involved this intriguing molecule.

6.1 Techniques which are routinely used in haemoglobin studies

6.1.1 Electrophoresis

Electrophoresis is a method of separating molecules from a mixture in solution by utilizing their electric charge. The amino acid side chains which protrude from the haemoglobin molecule are in many cases charged, and attract ions and cations to join with them. With changes in the pH of the surrounding medium, different groups of these side chains become electrically suppressed, leaving others unaffected. So the overall charge of the molecule changes with changing pH. Haemoglobin behaves as a Zwitter ion, being positively charged at the acid side of its iso-electric point, and negatively charged at the alkaline side. At its iso-electric point, the positive charges exactly equal the negative charges and the whole molecule is effectively uncharged. In the technique of electrophoresis the mixture of molecules is introduced to a buffer of a particular pH and the solution placed between electrodes. Provided the pH is not the isoelectric point of the protein, the charged molecules will slowly move either to anode or cathode.

Various supporting media are used in electrophoresis in order to stabilize the protein separation and permit recovery of the bands. Possibly the simplest involves the use of a strip of absorbent paper bridging the gap between electrodes, the sample being applied in the middle or at one end of the strip. Since some interaction between paper fibres and proteins does occur, rather better results are obtained using a more inert substance such as cellulose acetate. Of course most proteins are not coloured and cannot follow their movement during electrophoresis, but the red colour of haemoglobin makes it easy to follow its movement on the strip. If we wish to obtain better resolution of separate bands, and particularly to separate different haemoglobins from one another, then a porous gel will be the ideal choice of support media. The commonest are starch gels and polyacrylamide gels. In addition to the separating influence of the electric charges, such gels also act as molecular sieves, slowing down the progress of large molecules as compared to small ones. So gel electrophoresis exploits both size and charge of a molecule in executing its separation from others. Fig. 6–1 shows an example of haeomoglobins separated in this way, and a small polyacrylamide disc gel apparatus is both cheap to buy and fairly easy to run.

As with all scientific methods, caution is necessary in interpreting the results of electrophoretic protein separation. A single band following the

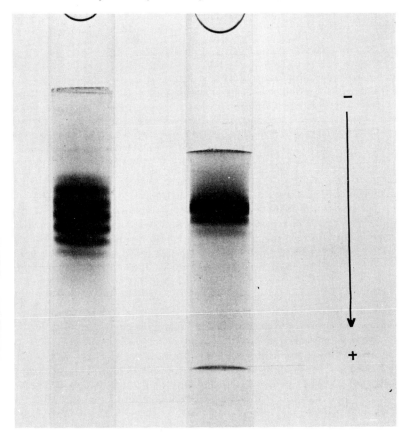

Fig. 6–1   Polyacrylamide electrophoresis of haemoglobins from two species of mullet fish.

electrophoretic run cannot necessarily be assumed to consist only of one protein species, since dissimilar molecules may migrate together at some or all pHs, and often repeated trials are necessary before an effective electrophoretic method can be found for separating two slightly dissimilar haemoglobins. On the other hand, separate bands do not always represent distinct protein species. Unless care is taken to avoid it, some proteins will polymerize and the polymers may band separately. Tetrameric molecules such as haemoglobin may also split into dimers and dimers produce spurious new bands. But, having stressed these possible complications, it must be emphasized that electrophoresis has proved a rapid and efficient way of routinely isolating many proteins.

6.1.2   *Chromatography*

The fundamental difference between chromatography and electrophoresis is that, in the former, the solvent liquid moves, carrying the molecules with it, whereas in the latter the solvent is stationary and the charged molecules move through it. If a drop of black ink is placed on a strip of absorbent paper and then one end of the strip is placed in a well of solvent, eventually the solvent front will pass through the drop. As the solvent continues to flow through and over the paper, different components of the ink flow forward at different rates, depending on their speed of movement through the paper and their solubility in the solvent. After a time bands of different colours can be detected, being the separate pigments used in the preparation of black ink. This is simple chromatography. As with electrophoresis, separation on paper is simple and easy but more sophisticated media yield better results. In particular, column chromatography involves filling a glass column with a mass of small water-saturated particles such as inert dextran. The sample is then introduced to the top of the column and the solvent allowed to flow through it. The column is porous and acts rather like a sponge. Very small particles will enter the orifices of the sponge and flow through the intra-sponge channels. Large particles cannot enter the sponge and so flow round it. In this way, large molecules flow through a column *quickly* and small molecules, by taking the long route through the column microchannels, flow slowly (see Fig. 6–2). This is the reverse situation to gel electrophoresis, where the gel is not truly porous, and small molecules move more rapidly than large.

An additional sophistication in column chromatography is provided by the use of ion exchange resins. These resins will bind proteins at some pHs, release them at others. So, following application of the sample to the top of the column, the buffer which is poured through the column is gradually altered to accomplish a slowly changing pH. Movement of a protein through the column depends both on its charge and its molecular size. In practice, the pH at which the starting buffer is employed is one at which the proteins will all bind to the column, and only as the pH changes

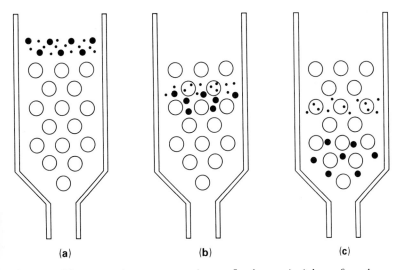

Fig. 6–2 Diagrammatic representation of the principle of column chromatography. Open circles represent swollen gel particles. Large and small dots represent large and small molecules. a, Mixture of molecules applied to column; b, large molecules starting to move ahead; c, large molecules leaving the column separated from small molecules. (Redrawn with permission of Dr. J. J. Marshall and Koch-Light Laboratories Ltd.)

are some proteins released to find their way through the column and out at the bottom where separation of buffer fractions is carried out.

6.1.3 *Fingerprinting of globins*

It is often necessary to compare or investigate haemoglobins more fundamentally than is possible by simple electrophoresis or chromatography. The ultimate chemical analysis of a haemoglobin tetramer must involve breaking it up into its constituent globins and then undertaking a study of the amino acid composition and sequence of each type of globin. I will now briefly describe how such an analysis is undertaken.

Firstly the isolated haemoglobin (recovered by prior electrophoresis or chromatography) must be reduced to globins and the haem groups discarded (since the haem group does not vary in differing haemoglobins it is of no interest in the analysis). This is accomplished by adding one volume of haemoglobin solution to some fifteen volumes of 1.5% HCl in acetone, cooled to 0°C. The globin appears in this solution, as a precipitate while the haem remains in solution, so centrifugation permits recovery of the globin free from haem. Following further washing of the globin in cold acetone (without HCl), the globin mixture can be studied. Very often the globin mixture may be analysed as a mixture, since most haemoglobins can be readily identified from the amino acid or peptide composition of the mixture. If the globins are to be studied separately they are dissolved in a buffer solution with a high concentration of urea and separated by electrophoresis in this buffer. The globins are not, of course, coloured, and their presence and position in the gel must be determined by staining. Whether in pure form or in a mixture, the globin preparation must now be itself further broken down or digested. This is done by using the enzyme trypsin. The enzyme hydrolyses the peptide bonds in the polypeptide chain wherever the amino acids lysine and arginine occur. The result of a tryptic digestion of globin is a mixture of peptides of varying sizes, ranging from two to thirty amino acids each.

We are now ready to undertake the actual fingerprinting. The peptides in the solution (which normally represent most but not necessarily the whole of the original globin) are evaporated to dryness and dissolved in a buffer ready for separation. The fingerprinting process consists of paper electrophoresis of the peptides, followed by paper chromatography, the second being carried out at right angles to the first. A large sheet of special paper is employed, the peptides being applied as a spot in one corner. The electrophoresis requires a very high voltage to obtain rapid and extensive spread along one end of the paper. After about one hour's electrophoresis the process is stopped, by which time a series of spots, each comprising a small number of different peptides, will be present along the appropriate edge. Chromatography is now carried out away from this edge, the solvent moving over the peptide spots and carrying them with it at rates depending on their solubility in it. After another few hours the chromatography can be stopped, the paper dried, and the task of visualizing each peptide undertaken. Some (those containing tryptophan) will fluoresce when the paper is placed under an ultra-violet lamp. The remaining peptides can be stained with ninhydrin, the actual colour produced being of some assistance in determining the amino acid composition of the peptides.

This two-dimensional pattern of peptides is the 'fingerprint' of the globin, and other globin preparations can be recognized as yielding the same or differing patterns. Although it is possible for proteins having, say, only one or two amino acid differences to yield the same fingerprint, in general the fingerprint pattern gives an accurate indication of identity and distinction in different globin preparations. A typical fingerprint pattern is shown in Fig. 6–3. If two globins are nearly identical in their patterns but have one peptide differently placed, this peptide may be eluted from the paper, hydrolysed with HCl, and subjected to amino acid analysis in a special apparatus termed an amino acid analyser. This is, in brief, the method by which the amino acid deviations in haemoglobins such as haemoglobin S have been determined.

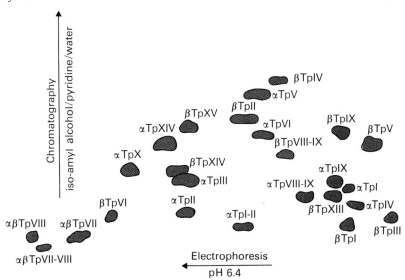

Fig. 6–3 Fingerprint of human haemoglobin A. αTpII indicates the tryptic peptide number two from the α globin chain. (From Lehmann, H. and Huntsman, R. G. *Man's Haemoglobins*. North Holland, 1974.)

6.2   Important experiments which involve haemoglobin

6.2.1   *Isolation and injection of globin messenger RNA*

If RNA is extracted from rabbit reticulocytes and run on a gel of soft acrylamide, a peak of RNA is recovered which has a sedimentation value of about 9S. Although many types of messenger RNA are found in most cells, with S values varying between 6 and 20S, globin message is present in great excess in reticulocytes and so yields a distinct peak of its own. The fact that this RNA is indeed the messenger RNA for globin has now been verified by its translation in a cell-free system, and the consequent production of globin. Globin mRNA was the first messenger RNA to be purified or identified and to date is the only one which can be isolated in bulk. Because of this fortunate availability, globin mRNA has come to be employed in a number of interesting experimental systems. I have already discussed in Chapter 4 the fascinating way in which radioactively labelled globin mRNA (or radioactively labelled globin DNA, transcribed from the globin mRNA by a viral reverse transcriptase enzyme) has been employed to localize the globin gene positions on chromosomes. We will now consider another group of equally exciting experiments utilizing globin mRNA, this time involving its injection into living oocytes. This work has been carried out extensively in the laboratory of Dr John Gurdon at Oxford and Cambridge.

The technique consists of the injection of globin mRNA into *Xenopus* oocytes or eggs by microsyringe. Rabbit globin mRNA was most frequently used, and its survival and effective translation was then monitored at intervals by searching for evidence of newly synthesized rabbit globin in the oocytes or developing *Xenopus* larva. The original experiments involved the use of unfertilized oocytes removed from the ovaries of female *Xenopus*. These cells can be retained in culture for some two weeks and so the provision of radioactive amino acids in the culture media ensures that the protein synthesized during culture will be radioactive. The injected message was faithfully translated in the oocytes, indicating that there is no species specificity governing cellular translational mechanisms.

The globin messenger RNA persisted in the oocytes throughout culture and competed with normal endogenous messages just as if it were normal *Xenopus* mRNA. The mRNA from both rabbit and mouse globin were tested and both gave rise to globin product with correct species characteristics. In addition, other types of mRNA, less readily available than globin mRNA but none the less procurable in small quantities from other laboratories, were also faithfully translated in the *Xenopus* oocyte. These injected mRNA types included those for mouse collagen, calf lens crystallin, trout testis protamine and honeybee promelletin.

Since oocytes are somewhat unusual cells with a restricted life in culture, it was of course extremely tempting to inject globin mRNA into fertilized eggs. This procedure poses greater problems than oocyte injection, and the first attempts yielded either dead embryos or ones which had cleaved very abnormally. These early difficulties have now been overcome, however, and both mouse and rabbit globin synthesis have been detected in the feeding tadpoles, indicating that the mRNA is as stable in the dividing cell situation as it had been in the non-dividing oocyte. This seems to demonstrate unequivocally that the injected message is not degraded or discarded. In addition, Gurdon has analysed the anatomical location of the added globin mRNA in the tadpole, and finds that, as determined by production of the appropriate globin, it is rather generally distributed and not restricted to tissues which would normally synthesize globin.

6.2.2   *Haemoglobin synthesis in erythroleukaemic cells*

A remarkable virus-induced leukaemia was discovered some years ago in certain strains of mice. It is termed Friend leukaemia after its discoverer. Some two weeks after a susceptible mouse is inoculated with the virus, it develops enlargement of the spleen and liver and acute erythroblastosis—that is great over-production of erythroblasts. The cells responsible for the leukaemia are lymphoid type cells, and they can be readily isolated and grown in culture.

Two important attributes of these leukaemic cell cultures deserve our attention. They are, firstly, that some of the cells in culture synthesize haemoglobin, underlining the fact that it is an over-production of lymphoid-type cells already in the erythroid compartment of differentiated cells, and secondly, that the synthesis of haemoglobin by these cells can be initiated or stimulated by exposing the cells to a substance called dimethyl sulphoxide (DMSO). There is good reason to think that this useful cell culture system will throw a lot of light on the process of erythroid differentiation.

6.2.3   Exploitation of the vertebrate erythrocyte nucleus

As mentioned earlier in this book, although the red blood cells of mammals are non-nucleated, those of lower vertebrates retain their nuclei. These nuclei are entire, and retain the full DNA complement of a normal diploid cell, but are relatively inactive in transcription. Indeed some, such as the nuclei of *Xenopus* erythrocytes, are entirely turned off. Such inactive nuclei provide excellent experimental material for those investigating the control of gene expression. Various laboratories have used such nuclei in different ways but I will only mention two particular lines of experimentation. The first consists of fusing these nuclei with growing cells of some other tissue and studying the reactivation of the erythrocyte nucleus. Professor Henry Harris at Oxford has exploited this system very fully, using chicken erythrocyte nuclei and rabbit macrophage or mouse fibroblast cells. The tissue cells are induced to engulf the nuclei into their own cytoplasm under the influence of an attenuated Sendai virus, the resulting cell coming to possess two nuclei each of a totally different kind (such a cell with two differing nuclei is termed a heterokaryon). Within such heterokaryons the chicken erythrocyte nucleus is found to become active and to initiate the production of some hen-specific protein.

A different approach, used largely in my own laboratory, is to utilize the isolated *Xenopus* erythrocyte nucleus as an example of complete genetic shutdown, and to attempt reactivation of some of its genes by presumptive regulatory proteins extracted from other cell types. The nuclei are first washed free from their own cytoplasm, then exposed in a suitable medium to the appropriate proteins, then again washed prior to being placed in a 'transcribing medium' of RNA polymerase enzyme and radio-labelled nucleotides. Whereas many cells do not yield proteins capable of inducing such reactivation, both the livers of young rats and the blood cells of highly anaemic *Xenopus* do, and column chromatography of such cytoplasm yields certain fractions which will reactivate nuclear transcription. Transcription in control batches of nuclei not exposed to such activating proteins is extremely low. By fractionating such presumptive regulatory proteins and analysing the RNA transcripts made in response to their activity, we hope to learn more about how genes are normally controlled within the cell.

Further Reading

Haemoglobin: structure, function and synthesis. *Br. med. Bull.* **32**, no. 3 (1976).

INGRAM, V. M. (1963). *The Haemoglobins in Genetics and Evolution.* Columbia University Press, New York.

LEHMANN, H. and HUNTSMAN, R. G. (1974). *Man's Haemoglobins.* 2nd edn. North Holland, Amsterdam.

MACLEAN, N. and JURD, R. D. (1972). The control of haemoglobin synthesis. *Biol. Rev.*, **47**, 393–437.

MACLEAN, N. (1976). *The Differentiation of Cells.* Arnold, London.

WEATHERALL, D. J. and CLEGG, J. B. (1972). *The Thalassaemia Syndromes.* 2nd edn. Blackwell, Oxford.

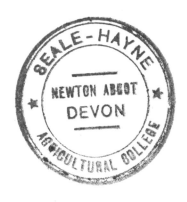